THE MOST AWKWARD PREGNANCY QUESTIONS ANSWERED!

Written By: Sam Hall

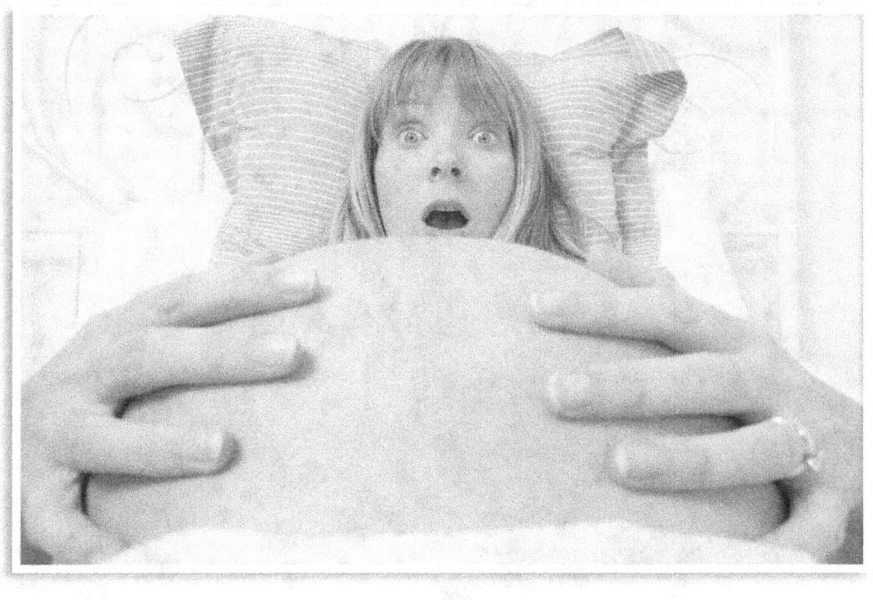

Pregnancy is a very unique and downright weird experience for your body to go through. After all, you are creating another human life. It's not always pretty, and someone who hasn't been through it has little reference to relate to you. Some of the things that your body is doing may be downright embarrassing, and hard to talk to your doctor about.

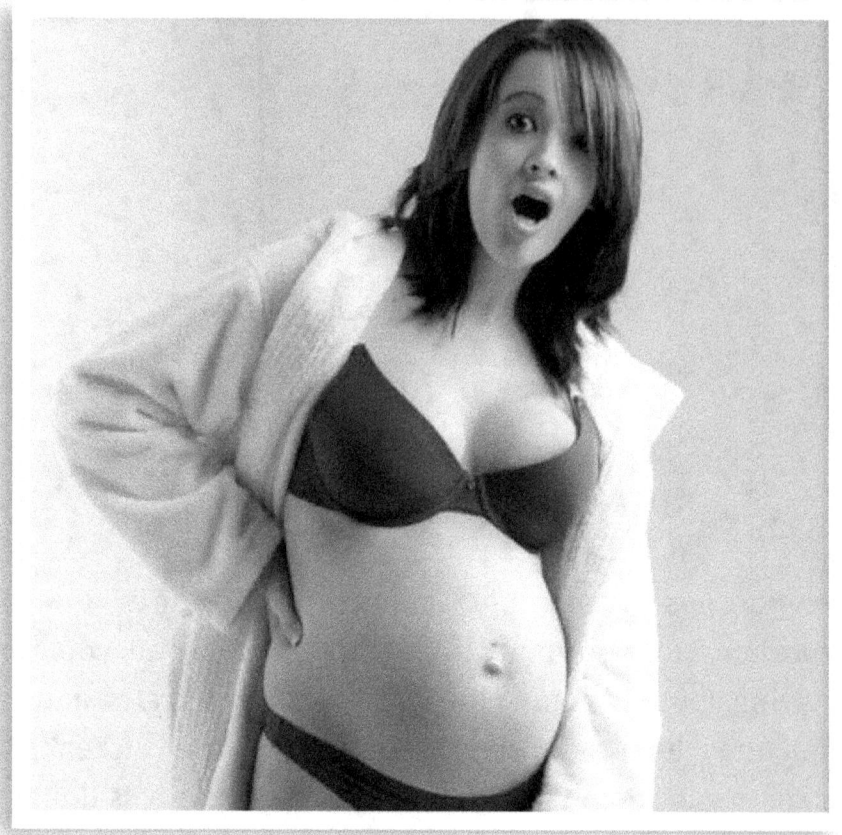

Don't worry, there's a plethora of weird and wonderful going on with your body right now, and that's perfectly normal and (mostly) temporary. From farts to discharge, sex to constipation, we've covered many of the most embarrassing questions you have about your pregnancy. So get ready for some real talk!

WHY AM I FARTING AND BURPING SO MUCH? IT'S DISGUSTING!

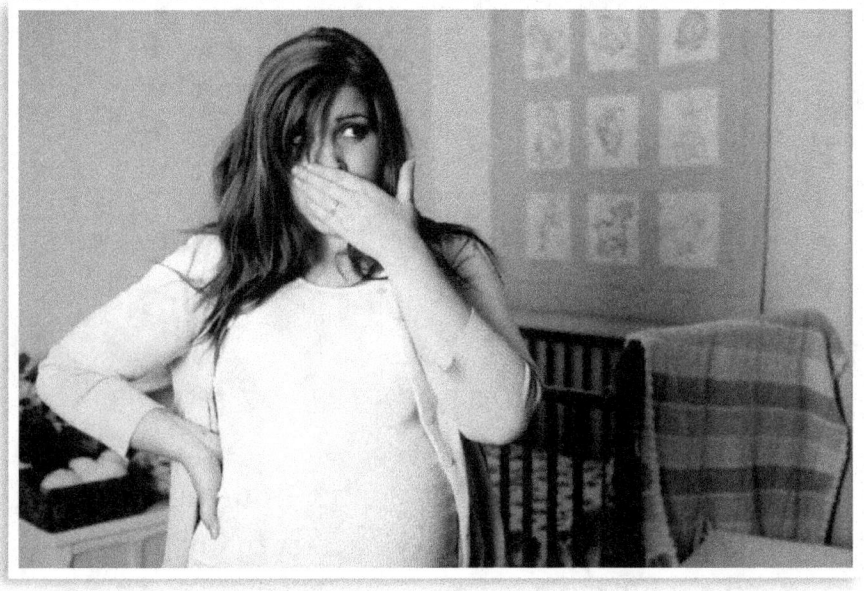

Alright, so now you're feeling some wicked gas at all times of the day, and whether it comes back up or travels on down there is little you can do to control it. Unfortunately, this is a natural effect of the crazy amount of rearranging your insides are doing to make room for baby. Also unfortunately, trying to hold it in can result in some pretty nasty ill effects. However, you're probably already making trips to the bathroom at least once an hour to empty your now tiny bladder, so take the time to let loose in the lou and the rest of the time you should be able to manage this.

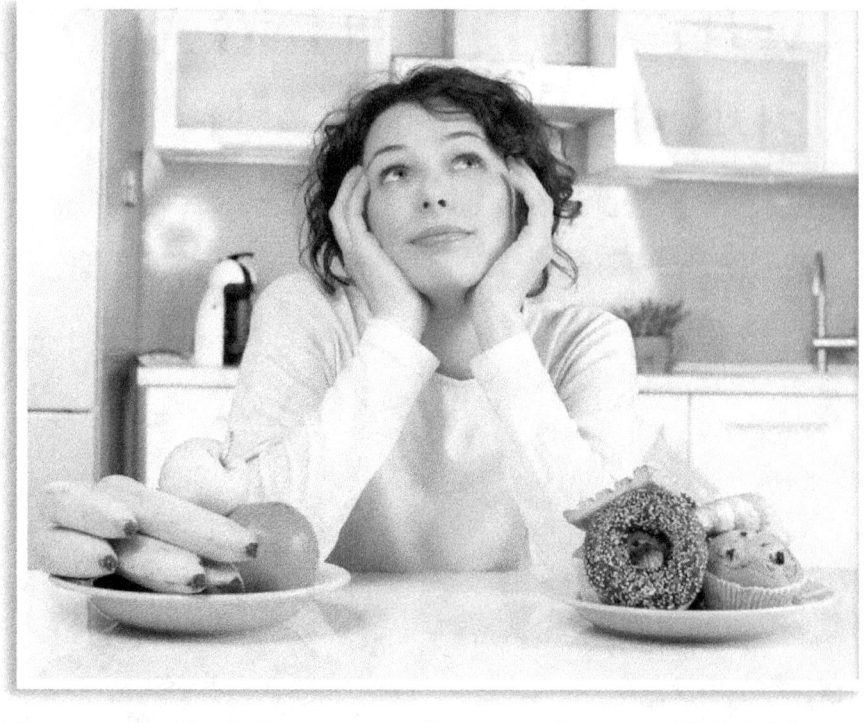

If you really find that you can't control yourself and it's becoming a problem, examine your diet to find out what foods you should cut back on. Spicy foods and musical fruits such as beans should be avoided, just make sure to replace them with other nutrient rich foods, and choosing to cut the grease and dairy (like ice cream) before you cut back on veggies.

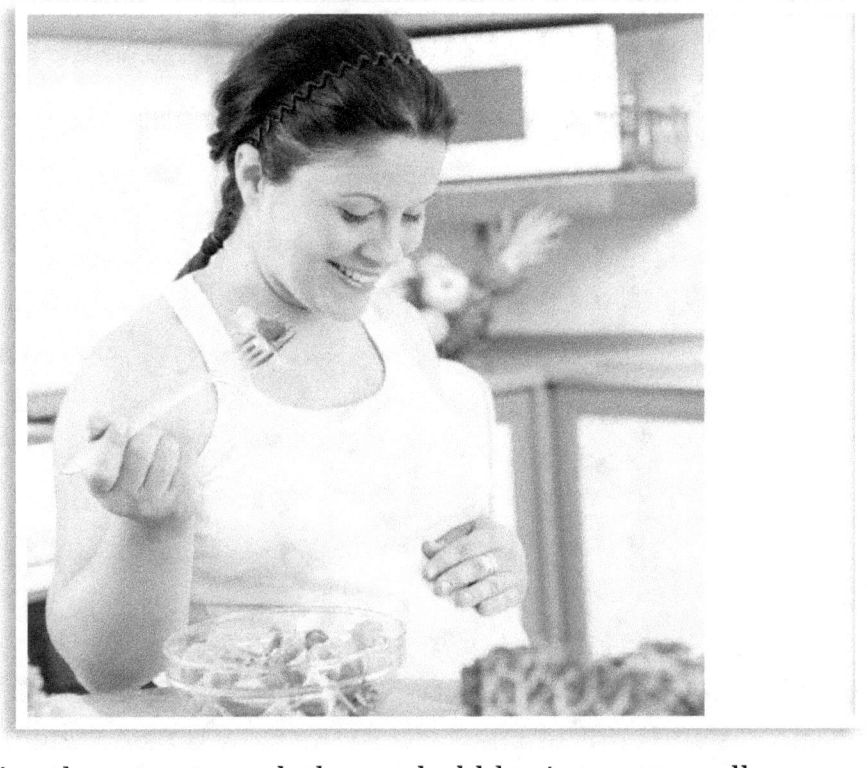

Another way to curb the gas bubbles is to eat smaller, more frequent meals (try 5 meals a day instead of 3), so that your digestive system has less to process at once. The bottom line is that there is no need to worry about excess gas, you're tummy's been going through a lot and has a right to complain.

WHY DO I HAVE HEMORRHOIDS?

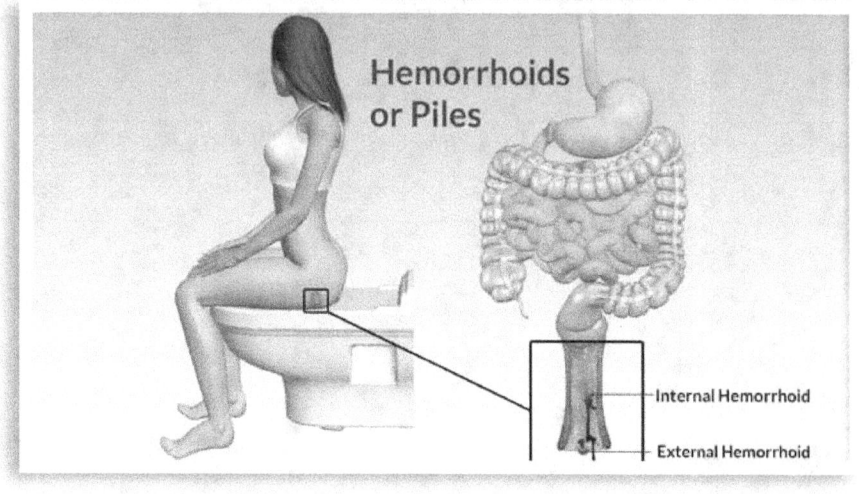

A combination of the common constipation pregnancy symptoms and additional pressure the baby puts on your veins during pregnancy may cause you to have hemorrhoids. These can be uncomfortable, and may even bleed from time to time. Even though hemorrhoids themselves are not cause for alarm, you need to tell your doctor about recurring blood in your stool so that they can rule out the minimal possibility of colon cancer.

SHOULD I BE WORRIED ABOUT HAVING SEX WITH MY PARTNER? WHAT'S SAFE?

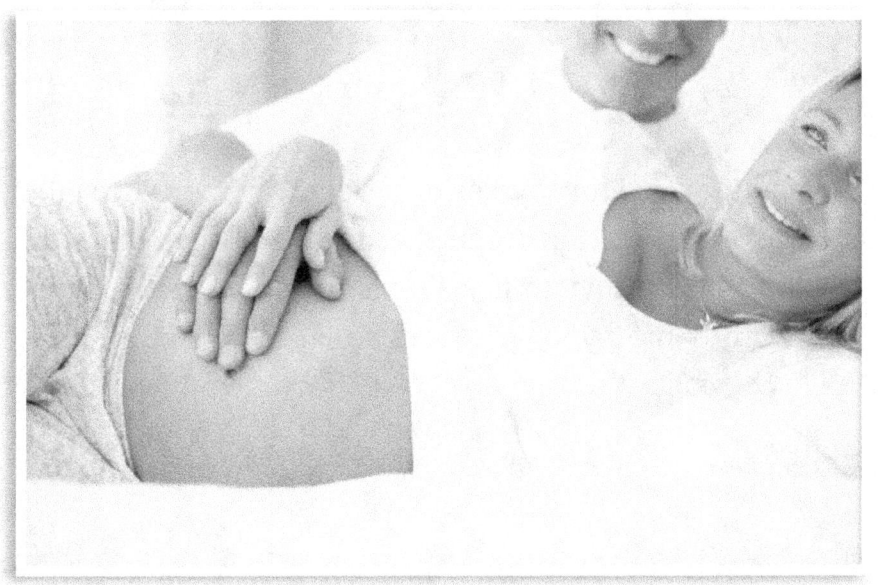

The good news is, sex in general is safe and healthy during pregnancy. You may have to modify your positions for comfort, but otherwise your doctor will tell you if there are special concerns regarding the need for "pelvic rest" (aka, don't go there). Of course, if you feel any pain during intercourse it's best to dial it back and speak to your doctor on your next visit.

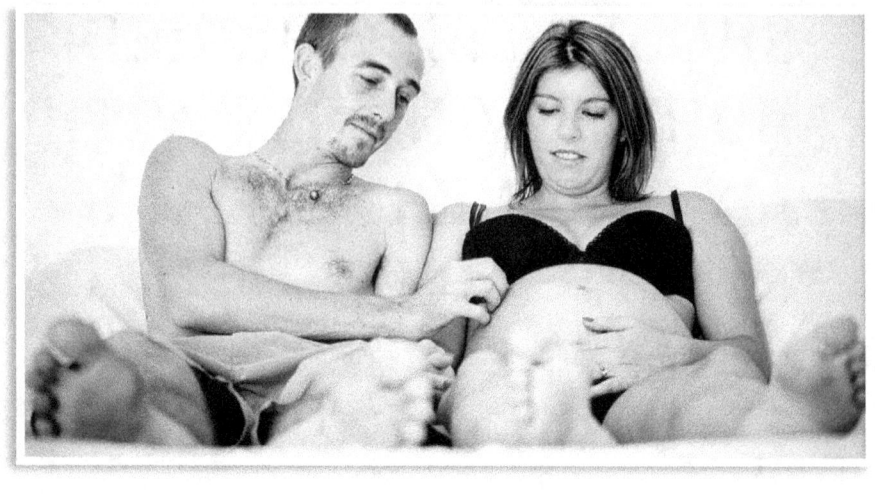

Later on in your journey, sex is a great way to induce labor, as there are chemicals in the sperm called prostaglandins, which can help move things along. Around week 39, you may want to jump your partners bones a few extra times due to this fact.

CAN I USE BY VIBRATOR DURING PREGNANCY?

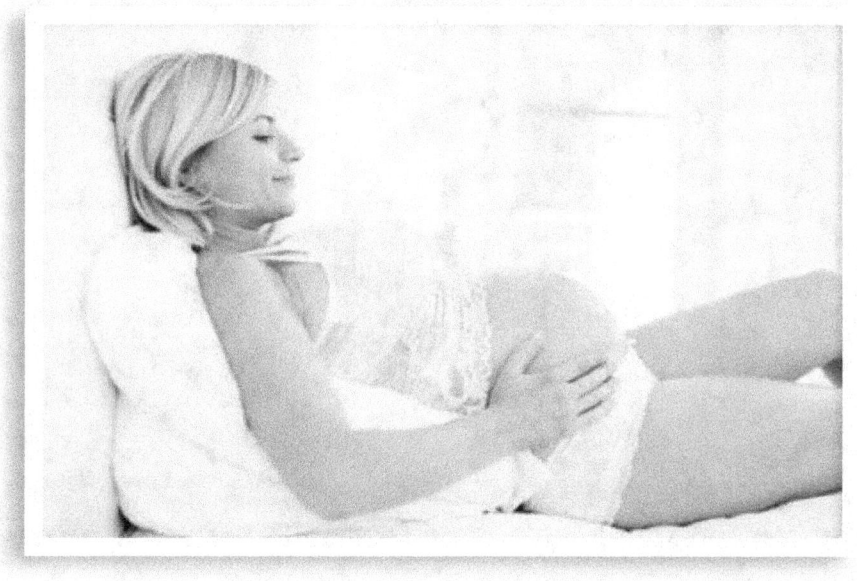

Just like sex, your favorite sex toys are generally approved pastimes during pregnancy. Make sure that anything (including your partner) that you put up there is clean and sanitary, and don't use anything too elaborate that could go beyond your cervix, and you should be fine. Again, any pain you feel should be reported to your doctor before you go for a repeat performance.

WHAT ABOUT ORAL SEX?

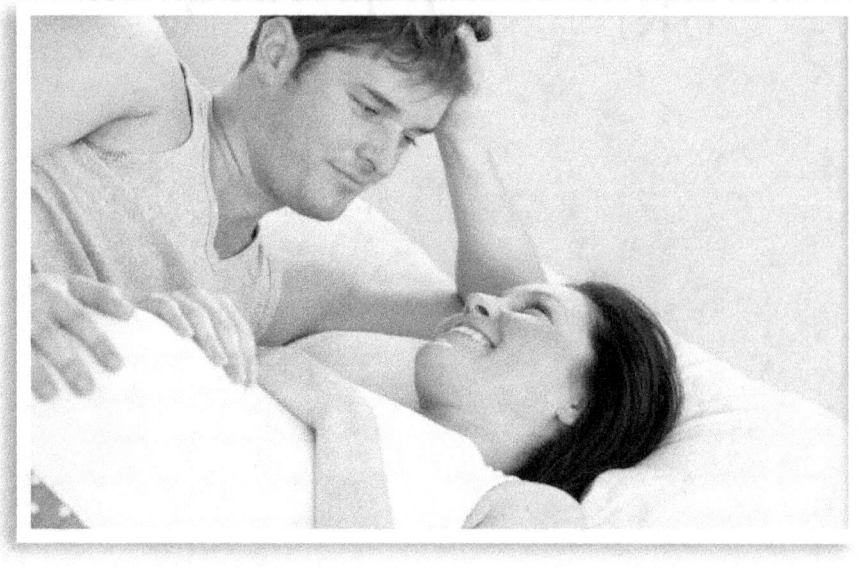

You can and should enjoy oral sex at all times, even during pregnancy. Additional foreplay can pave the way for a great experience even when you've got positional limitations as in the third trimester. It's also a great way to warm up to prevent the necessity of lubricant, which some women may find irritating on sensitive pregnancy skin. So, give it a go!

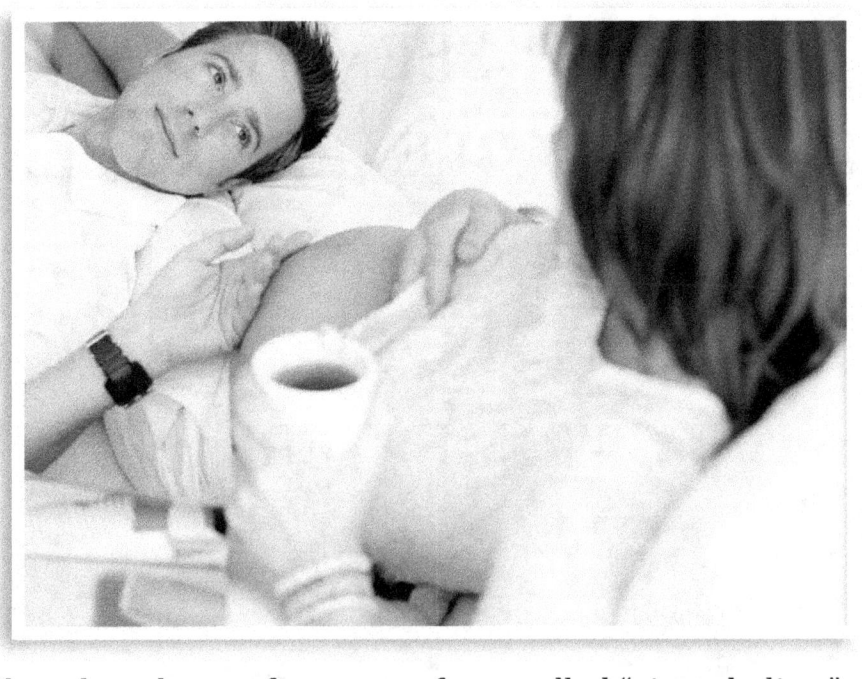

There have been a few cases of a so-called "air embolism" occurring when a partner forcibly blows air directly into the vagina. These cases are extremely rare, but if you're concerned lay down an air-free ground rule prior to laying back and enjoying.

I CAN'T SEEM TO GET COMFORTABLE DURING SEX. IS THERE A BETTER POSITION FOR THIRD TRIMESTER?

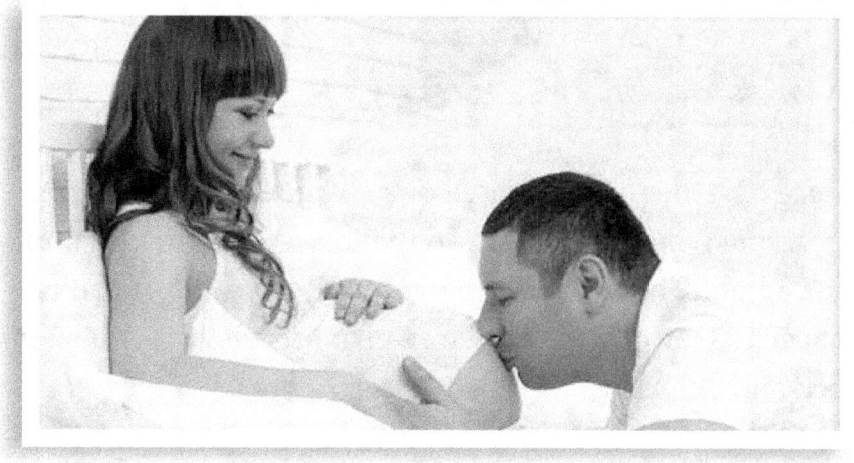

Pressure on the belly can be extremely uncomfortable during intercourse in the third trimester, which can make having sex difficult. Try a side by side approach, or get on top. You may require some extra props and pillows to make things work for you. Pro tip: break out your yoga ball as a support.

I DON'T WANT TO HAVE SEX AT ALL ANYMORE. WHAT'S WRONG WITH ME?

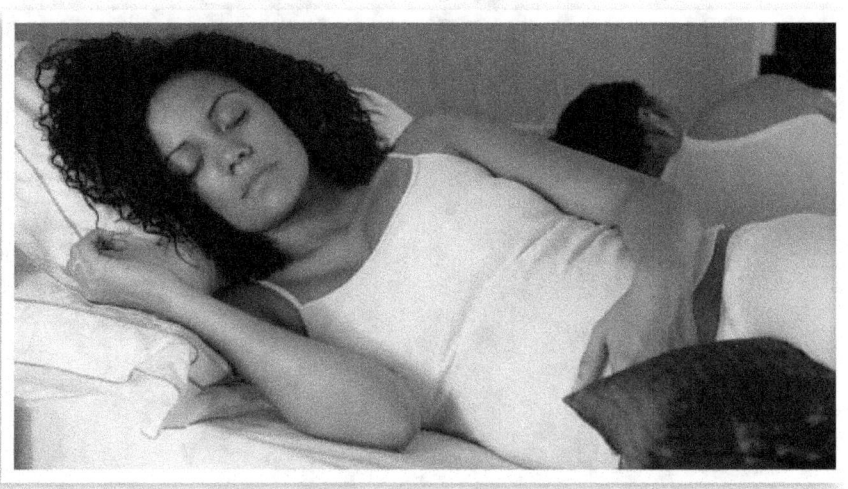

Pregnancy hormones can wreak havoc on your sex drive, which can be a real bummer for your partner. In fact, the large majority of women report feeling uninterested in sex at some point during their pregnancy. Many later report a huge upswing in libido in the second or third trimester, but if this doesn't happen to you don't worry. Keep your partner in the loop and make sure to address things with your doctor if it begins to interfere with your relationship.

I'M SO RANDY LATELY, I CAN'T GET ENOUGH SEX!

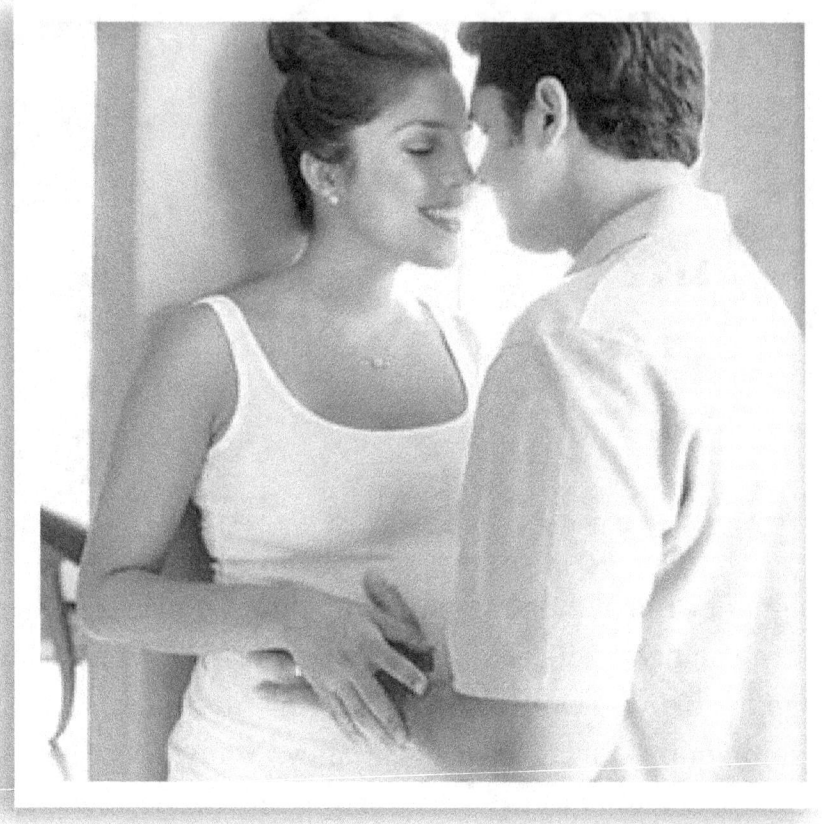

On the other end of the spectrum, sometimes your hormones will take a nice upswing. Many women report a period of their pregnancy when sex becomes extremely enjoyable. All I can say is, get it girl!

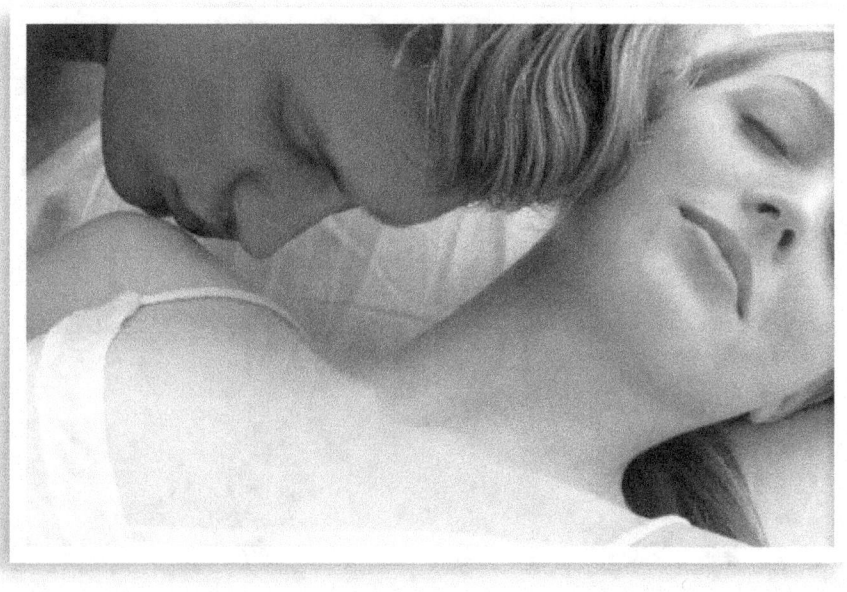

You can also feel discomfort and pressure in your pelvis as the baby drops, which can limit the depth of penetration that is comfortable for you. Modify your positions and incorporate some more foreplay to make the experience more enjoyable for both parties.

WILL MY HUSBAND STILL WANT TO HAVE SEX WITH ME AFTER WITNESSING THE BIRTH?

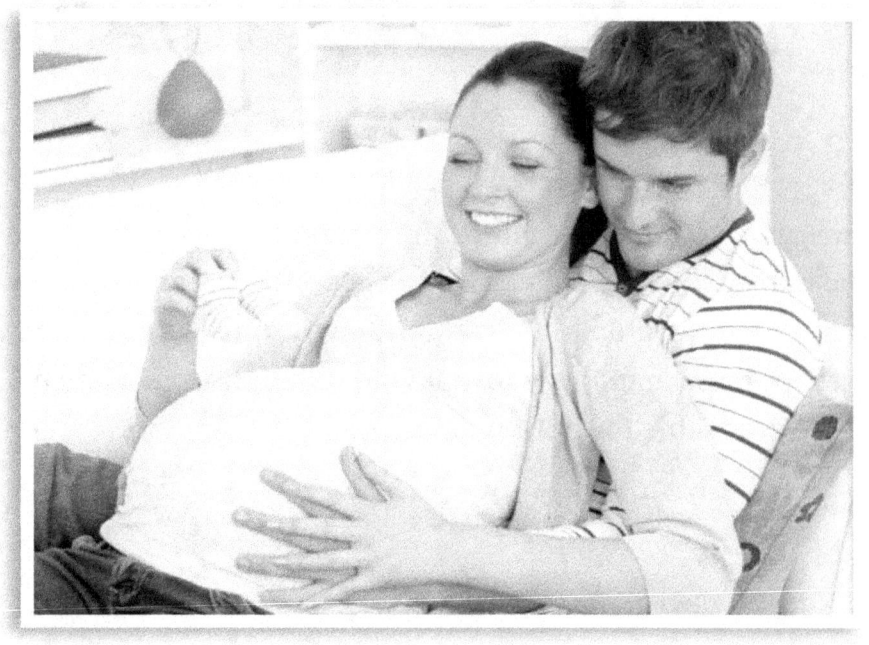

The answer is yes, of course he will. This is one of those pregnancy anxieties that can get the best of us, but really has little merit. You are bringing his child into this world, after all, and he knows how that works (if not, it's time to do a little youtube search and educate your man). Besides, you won't want to let him anywhere near your naughty bits while they are healing, likely 6-8 weeks after the delivery date. By that time, he'll be very ready to do the deed.

WHY CAN'T I POOP?

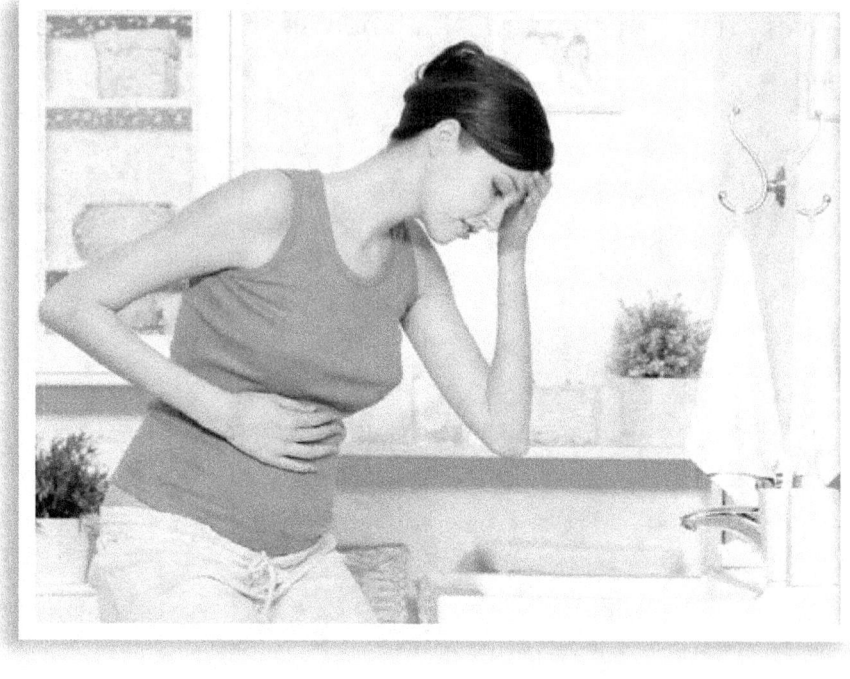

A combination of hormones and your compressed insides are to blame for this very annoying and often painful pregnancy symptom: constipation. Around half of all women experience it during some point in their pregnancy, though knowing you're not alone isn't the most comforting prospect when you're bent over in the lou.

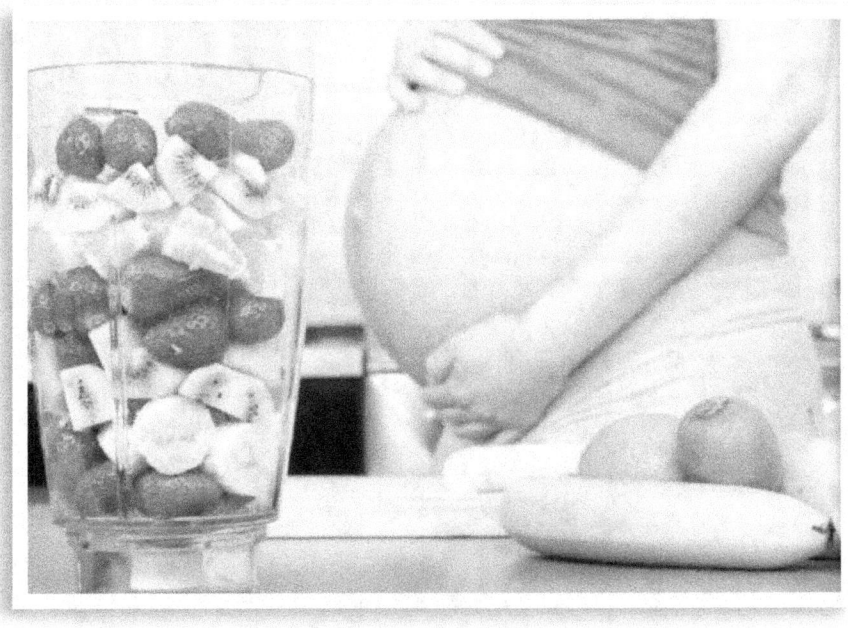

Grab yourself some extra fiber, and try to manage it through diet. Moderate exercise may also help, so grab your trainers and head out for a walk around the block. Drink an extra glass of water or two. Whatever you do, make sure that you consult your doctor before resorting to any sort of over the counter medication, as these can leave you dehydrated and depleted, neither of which are good for your little one.

WHY DO I LEAK ALL OF THE TIME?

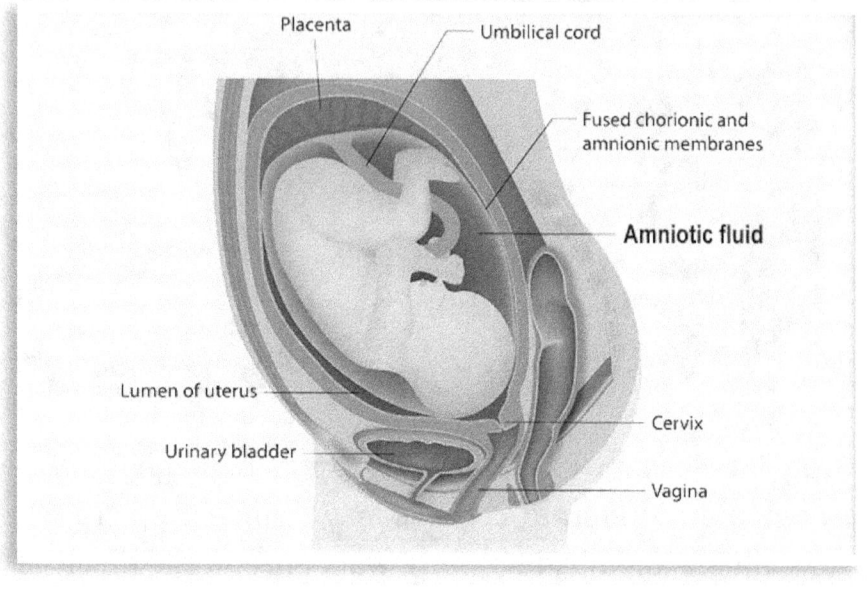

Bladder leakage, especially when coughing, sneezing, or laughing, is the most prevalent and also most annoying of all pregnancy symptoms. Pressure on your bladder and urethra from your uterus' new position as well as the growth of your little cherub are to blame. It doesn't help that you are gulping down way more water to keep things moving and stay cool.

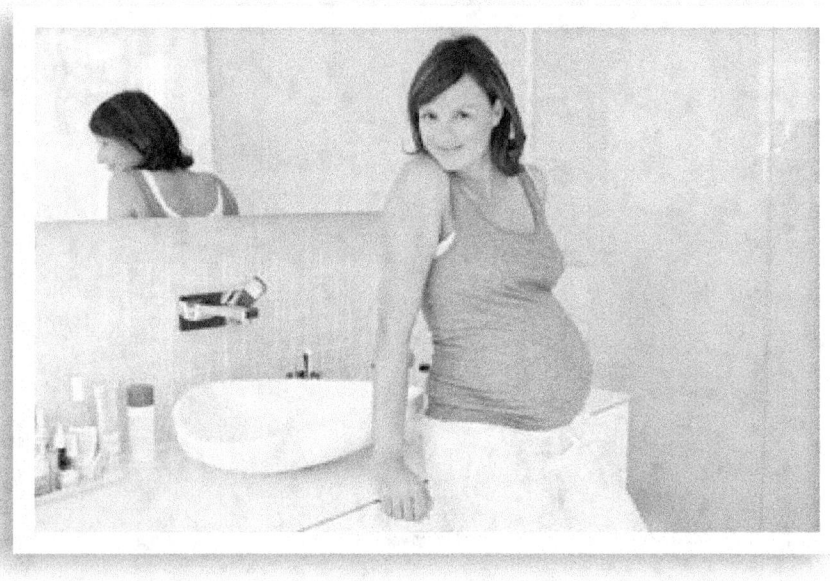

The best way to cope is to manage your trips to the bathroom, simply so that there is less there to leak. Be sure that you are headed there each time you feel the urge to pee, for a random sneeze could come at any time. Set a timer on your phone, so that you visit the lou at least once an hour, and you may find that this takes care of itself.

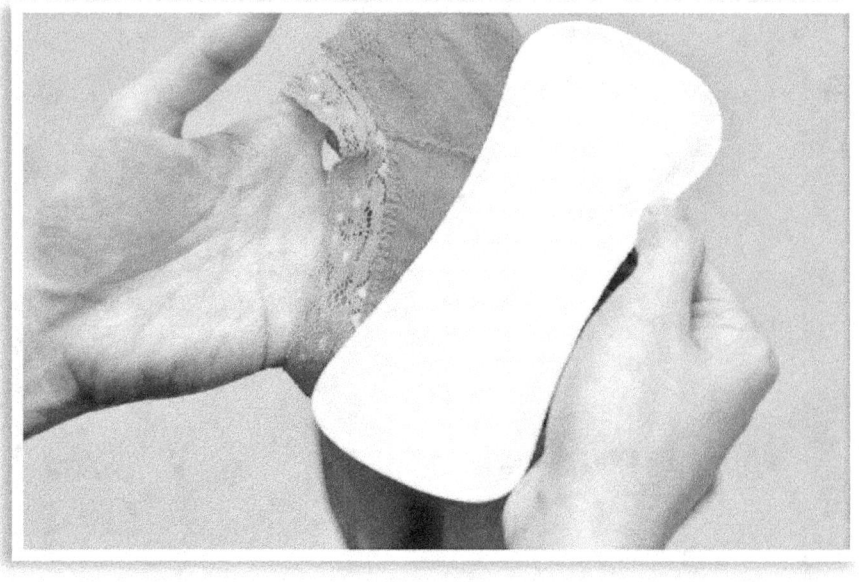

If you still have some rogue drips and dribbles, grab a sanitary napkin and wear it when you're away from an extra change of drawers. It's not foolproof or the most comfortable of solutions, but it's probably better than walking around with a urine spot on your pants for all to see.

I SEEM TO HAVE A LOT OF VAGINAL DISCHARGE, MUCH MORE THAN NORMAL

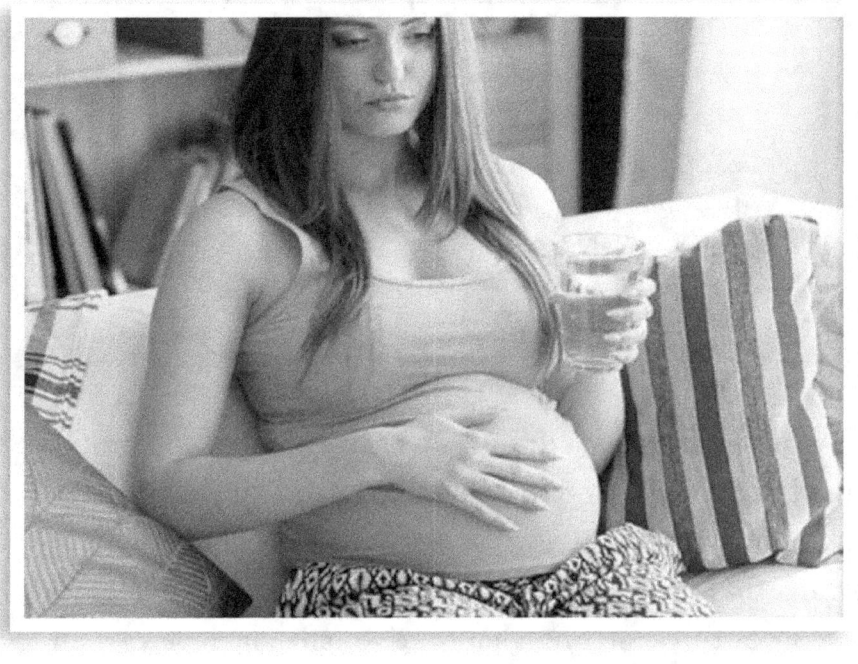

Your body kicks a lot of defense mechanisms into high gear when you're making a baby, and this is one of them. In order to purge bacteria and other nasties away from your adorable one, your vagina will up its discharge game.

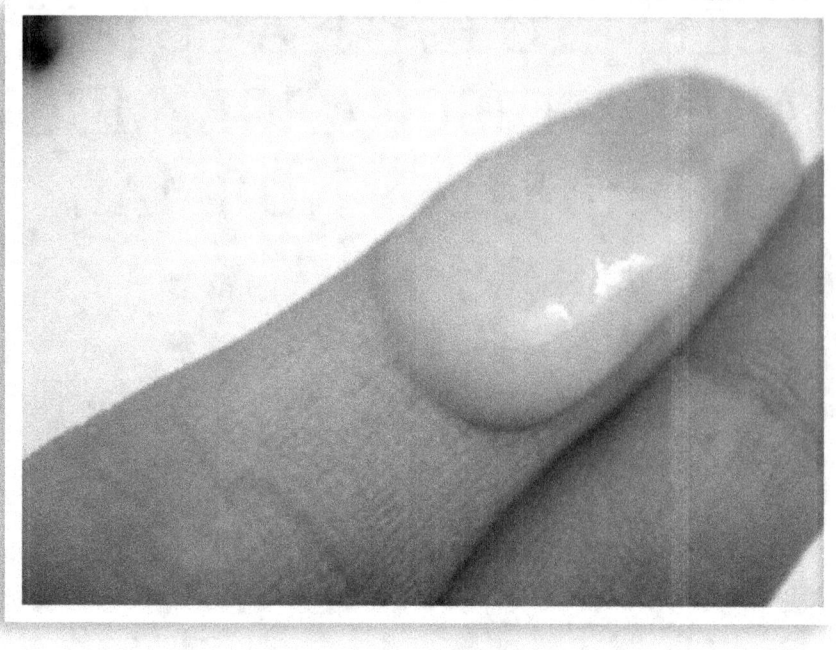

There's no 'normal' amount for this nonsense, so you may just have to get used to some extra rinsing for your laundry. Think of it as practice for all of the wonderful stains that are in your future. However, if the discharge becomes thick, strongly colored, burns, or develops an order, get checked for an infection by your practitioner ASAP.

I'VE NOTICED SOME OTHER CHANGES.. DOWN THERE

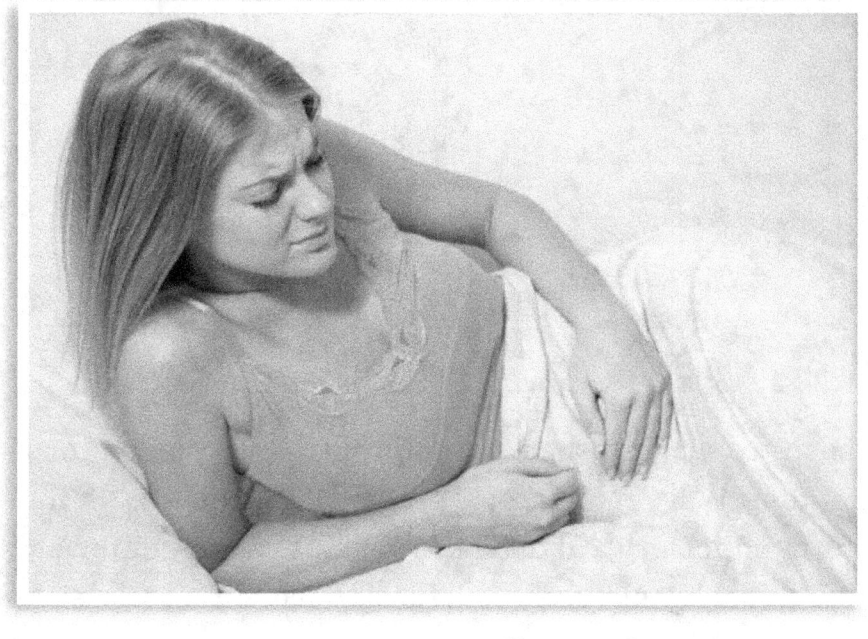

Many pregnant women report swelling and sensitivity changes in their lady parts during pregnancy, especially in the third trimester. You may also feel pressure from the baby dropping into the pelvis in preparation for birth. None of these symptoms are cause for alarm, unless they cause you extreme or persistent discomfort.

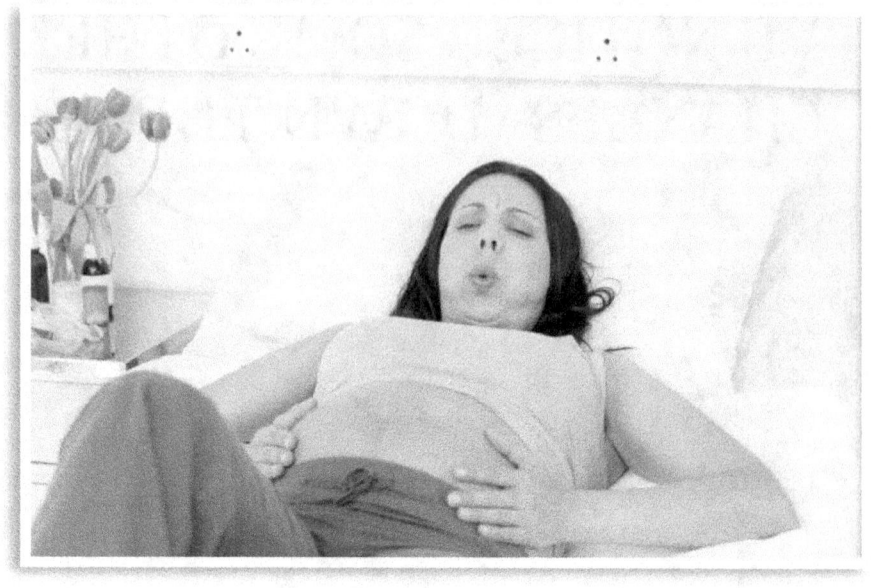

Sharp groin pain, especially upon changing positions or standing, is a common early pregnancy symptom. As your uterus shifts forward to make room for baby, your lower abdominal ligaments stretch beyond what they've ever experienced before. Take a load off and wait for it to pass.

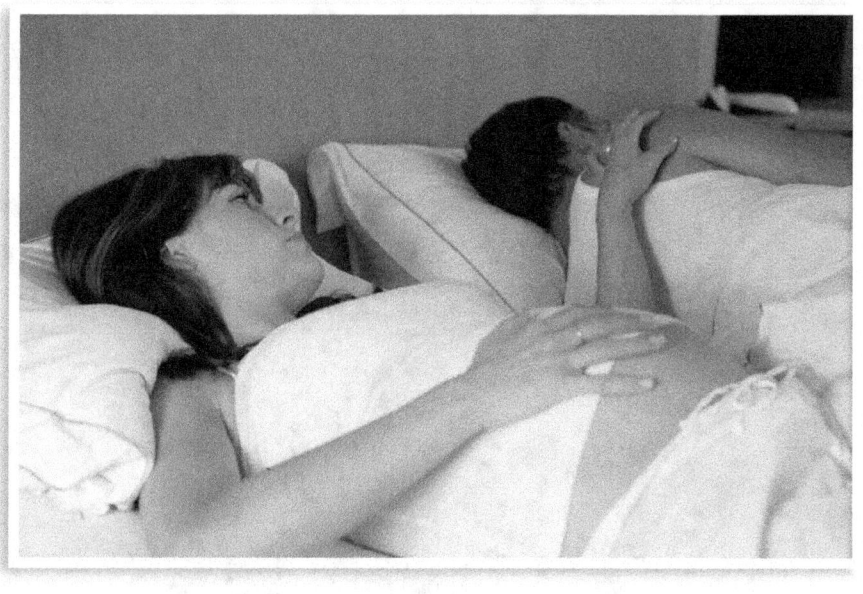

Later on, pain in your groin can be caused by baby dropping into the birthing position, or Braxton-Hicks contractions. These are both normal, but if you notice contractions that are persistent, increase in pain, or increase in frequency, give your doc a call.

I HAVE SWOLLEN VEINS ON MY LADY PARTS!

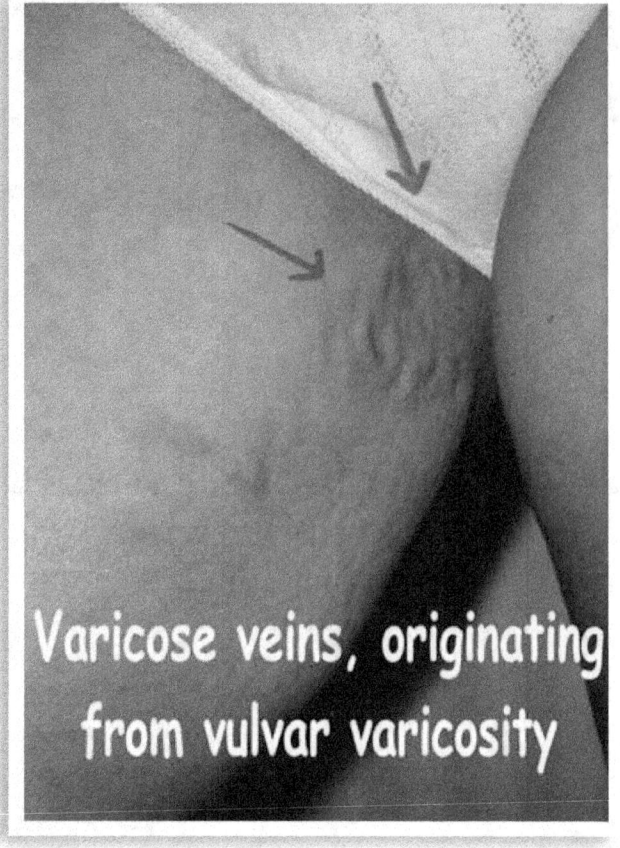

Varicose veins, originating from vulvar varicosity

Vulvar varicose veins, as they are known, can be caused by the same factor that contributes to hemorrhoids: pressure of your growing uterus on the vascular system down there. Unlike hemorrhoids, however, they will not open up and bleed. Even better: they will likely disappear very soon after birth.

I'M HAVING VERY STRANGE DREAMS. IS THIS NORMAL?

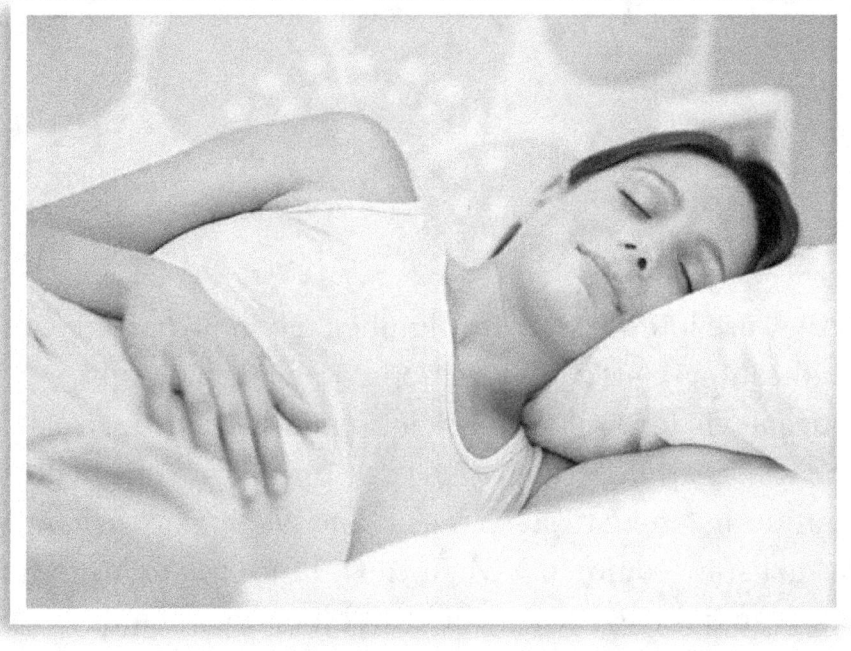

In a word: yes. Pregnant women report all kinds of vivid dreams, from the sexy to the sinister. One explanation is hormones, another is the shear amount of new information your subconscious mind is trying to process in advance of this big change. As long as your dreams aren't interfering with your rest, just go with it.

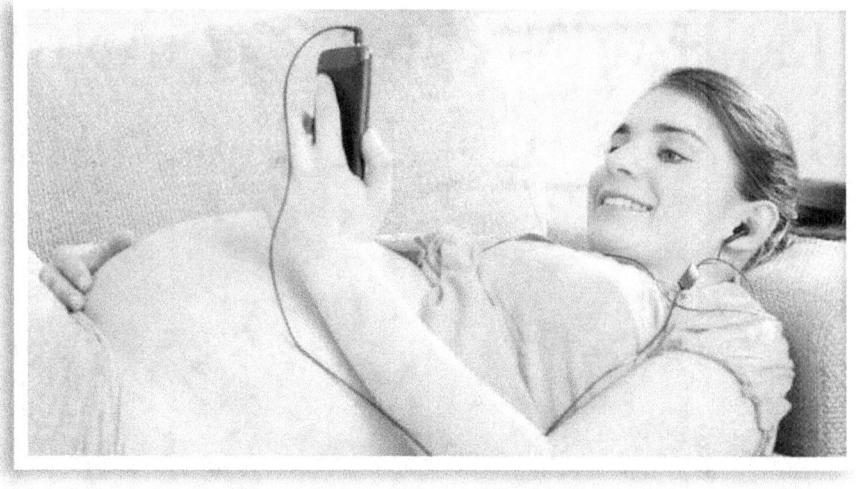

If they are interfering with slumber, try some non-medication related interventions. Keeping a dream journal will let you look back later and see the fun. You can also try things such as sticking to your normal bedtime routine, listening to sleep music, and writing down your to-do list for tomorrow when you hit the sack to make sure your mind is clear when you drift off to dreamland.

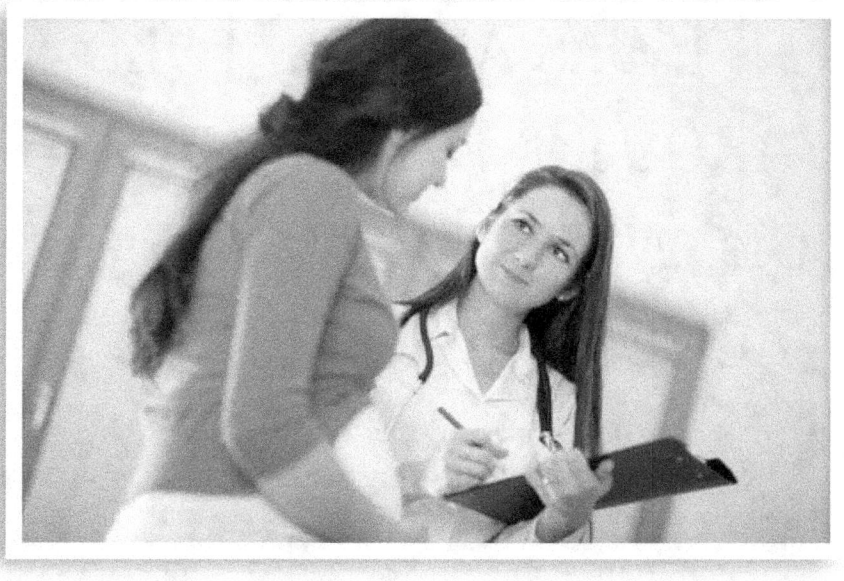

In extreme cases, your doctor may prescribe a sleep aid that is safe for you to use during pregnancy. Make sure to follow the advice on the prescription. This usually involves taking the medication only when you are ready for sleep, and don't wait until you only have 4 hours left before you need to get out of bed.

I WAS ALWAYS TOLD ABOUT THE PREGNANCY 'GLOW', BUT NOW I'VE GOT ACNE LIKE A TEENAGER!

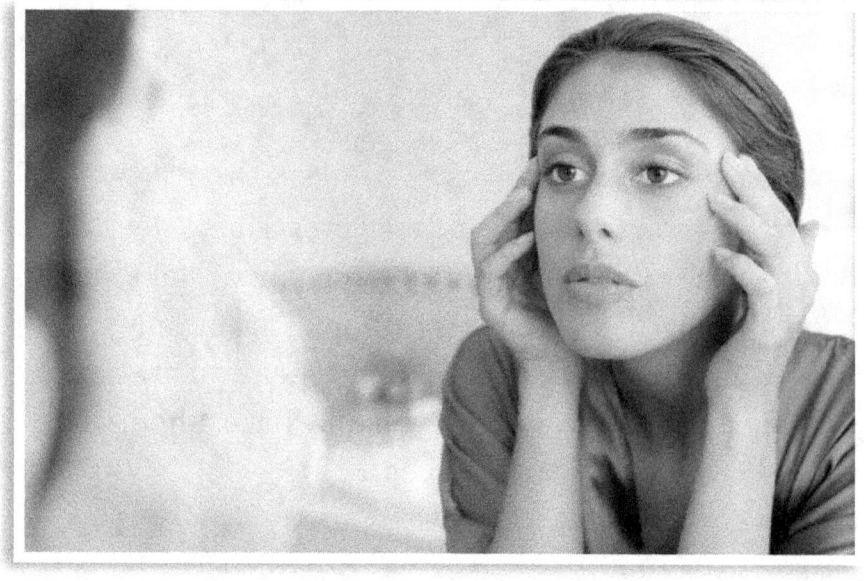

Yes, the romanticized versions of pregnancy that we cling to when trying to conceive are often very unrealistic. People around us and idyllic celebrity pregnancies feed into this. However,while increased blood flow can give your skin a nice glow, your hormonal changes are likely wreaking havoc on your complexion in a variety of ways.

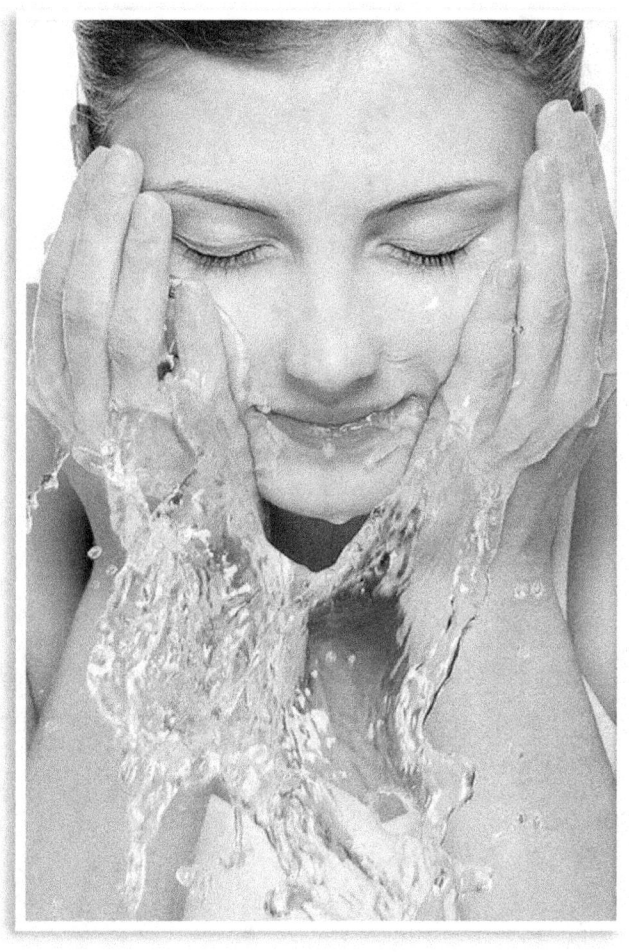

Try the old teenager tricks of cutting down on greasy foods and excess sweets, and make sure you are washing your face regularly especially before bedtime. Freshly laundered pillowcases will also help keep bacteria at bay. You should avoid switching to a harsher facial wash, and stick with something mild. After all, your skin is more sensitive during pregnancy. Besides, the main culprit is hormonal, which is more of a wait-it-out prospect.

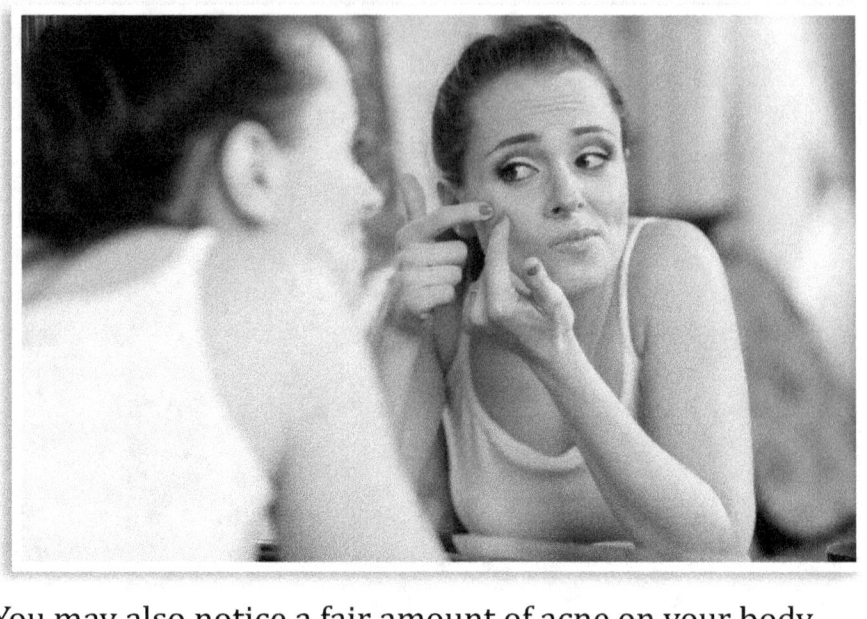

You may also notice a fair amount of acne on your body. Use the same tips above and avoid switching to a harsher body wash. Just add it to the list of reason's you're going to teach that little one to help you with the chores as soon as they learn to walk.

THERE ARE LITTLE SKIN TAGS POPPING UP ALL OVER THE PLACE... WHAT GIVES?

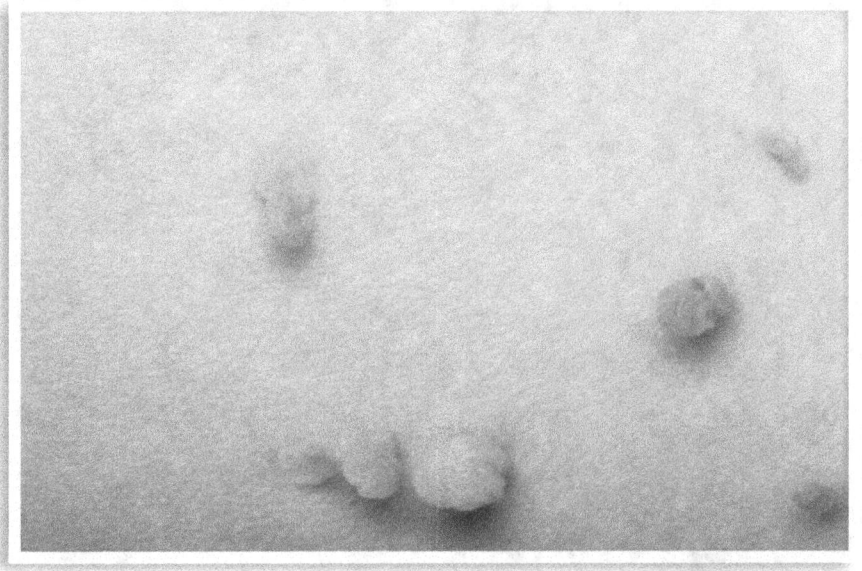

Among the myriad of skin related symptoms no one told you about, you may have little bits of skin popping up. These can be caused by a combination of cell-preserving hormones and friction with clothing. Don't fret, these will disappear as well when your hormones return to normal.

WHAT IS THIS DARK LINE ON MY BELLY?

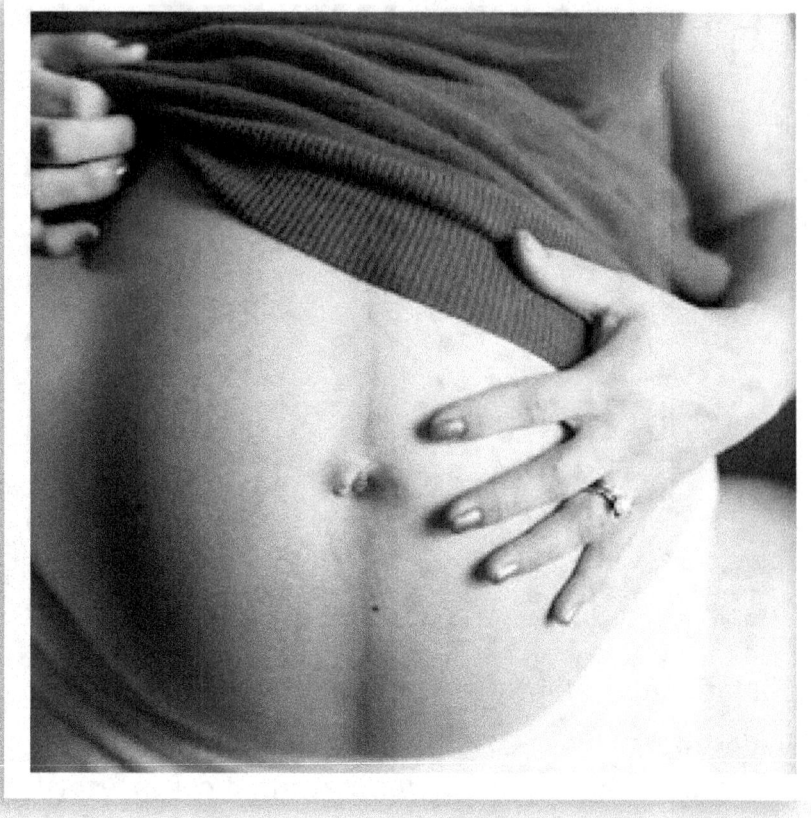

Linea Negra, or a darker line down the middle of the lower part of the belly, occurs in roughly ⅓ of pregnant ladies. Its presence may become more apparent with sun exposure, so cover up if you're concerned. The pigment change is not permanent, so relax.

I'M SEEING RED SPLOTCHES ALL OVER, EVEN ON MY FACE?!

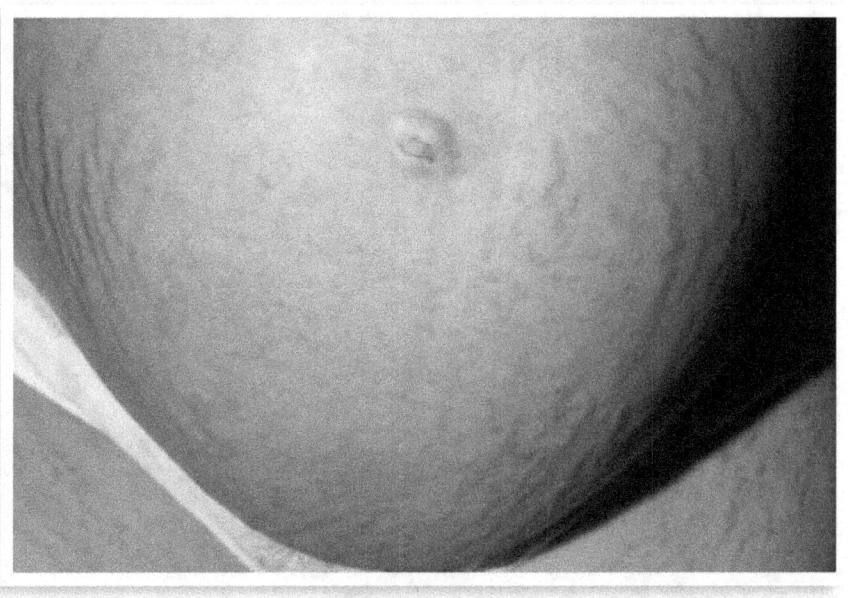

Your body's hormones are increasing your production of melanin, which can give you some odd skin decorations. Again, this can be exacerbated by sun exposure, so cover up as best you can. Talk to your doc about anything that you are concerned about, but for the most part your hormones will go back to normal, taking the extra melanin with them.

I HAVE HAIR IN ALL KINDS OF PLACES I'VE NEVER HAD ANY BEFORE... WHAT'S WRONG WITH ME?

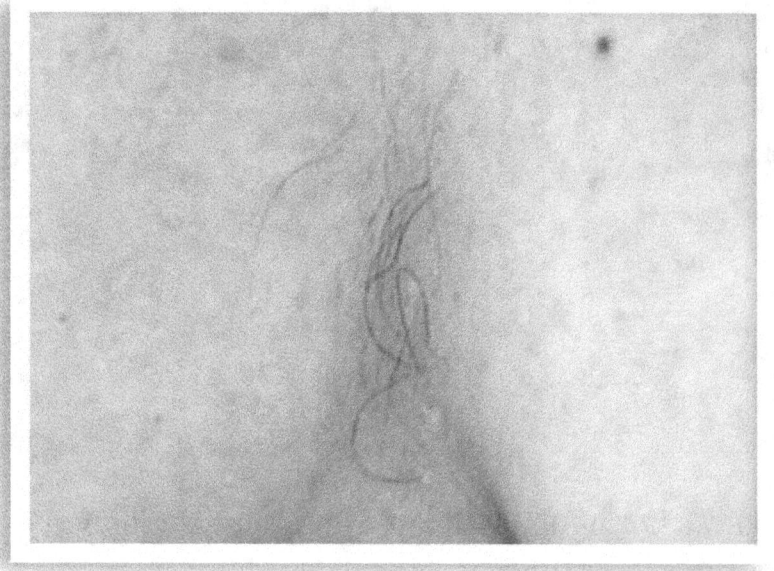

Happy pregnancy hormones to you! Many women report thicker hair popping up on their arms, legs, face, and breasts at various times during pregnancy. This is completely normal. Even better: when your hormone levels return to normal, so will your body hair. Break out the razor and tweezers if it bothers you, and know that this too shall pass.

CAN I GET A BIKINI WAX WHILE PREGNANT?

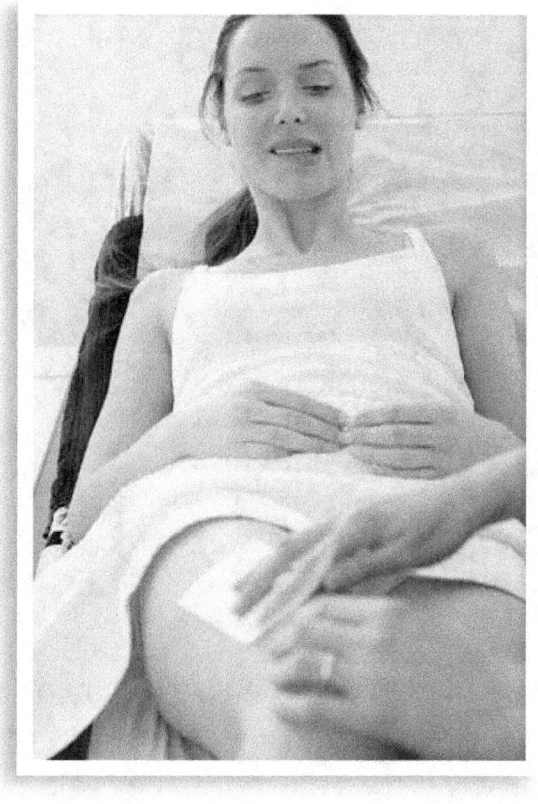

Generally practitioner's don't have a problem with waxing your outer body. But, be warned: your sensitive skin may make this procedure much more painful than the last time you were at the salon. It's a good rule of thumb to avoid chemical hair removal lotions and laser hair removal treatments during pregnancy for this very reason.

WHY ARE MY NIPPLES ITCHY?

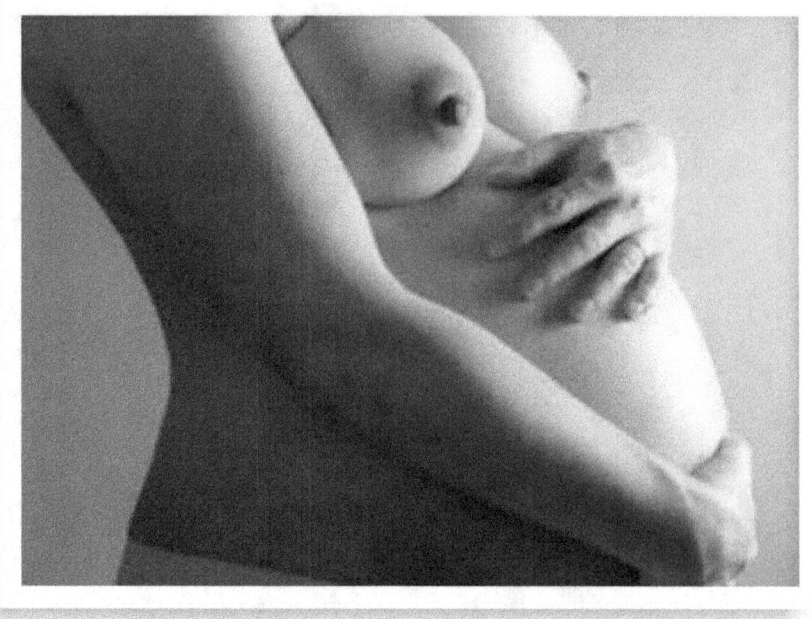

Nipple changes, and breast changes in general, can be a jarring reality for pregnant women. As your breasts prepare themselves for a newborn, they gain tissue mass and the nipples can expand and darken. One of the best ways to combat the itch, not just on your nipples but all over, is to moisturize. There are nipple creams on the market, but for now your normal lotions or cocoa butter should suffice. Spread it on after a shower to get as much benefit as possible.

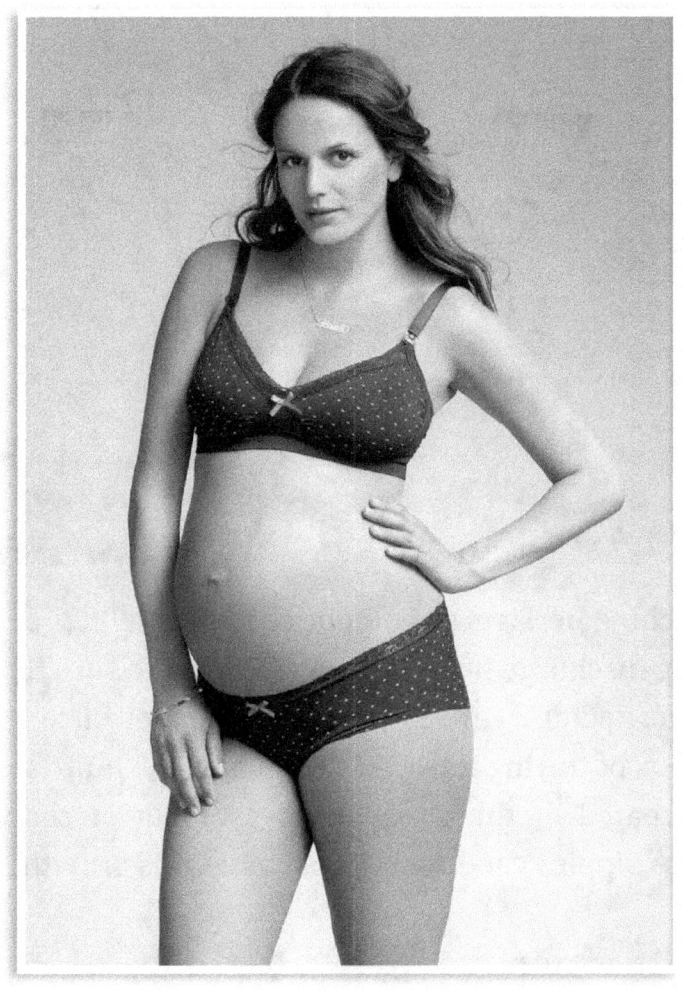

You may also take this opportunity to reevaluate your brassiere situation. If you haven't tried on a larger bra in a while, grab your purse and head to the store. Your mams will thank you when they have enough room to breathe.

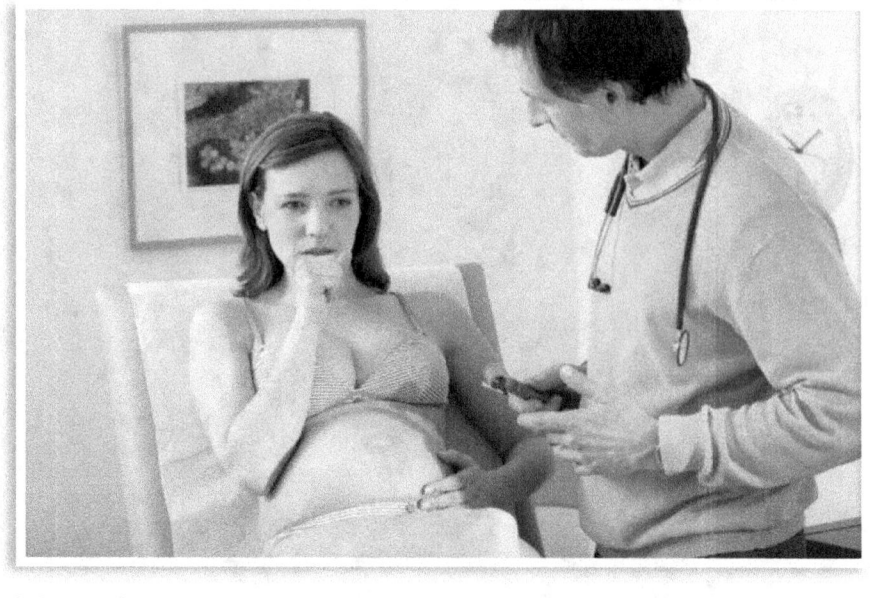

If the itching persists or you notice green, yellow, or foul smelling discharge from your nipples, make sure that you give your doctor a call. Rarely women experience infections of the breasts, which can become quite serious if left untreated. In the rarest of cases, bloody discharge from the nipples can be a sign of cancerous growth.

WHY ARE MY NIPPLES LEAKING?

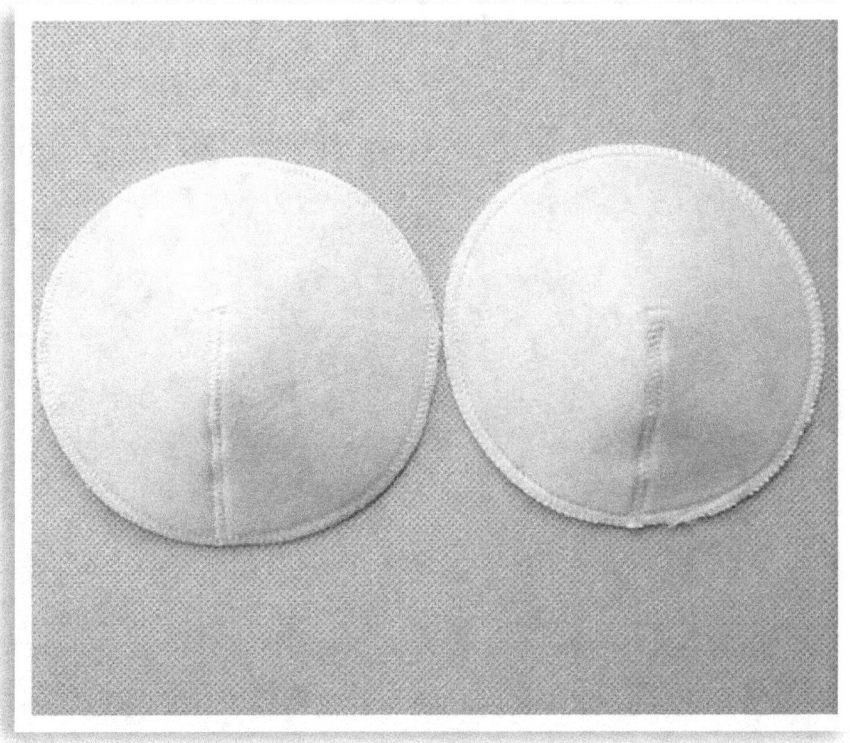

Your breasts are changing in many ways, all to prepare for the functional feeding purpose that they were designed for. Toward the end of pregnancy, this may cause your nipples to leak a little bit. Mention it to your doctor, but it is usually nothing to worry about. You can buy nursing pads to place in your bra to save your clothes. Do report any color or odor changes in the discharge though, as this may be an indication of infection.

HOW DO I HANDLE VOMITING EVERYWHERE I GO?

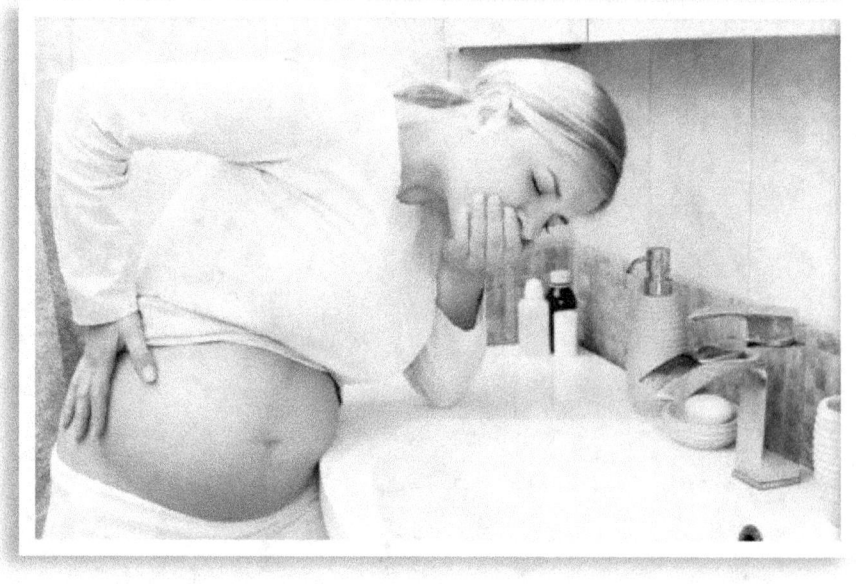

It may sound cheeky, but carry a bag and some tissues with you to wipe your mouth. Some mints wouldn't be a bad idea either. You can look into the various ways to cope with the ineptly named "morning" sickness, and find which ones work for you. If nothing works, discuss it with your doctor, but know that by the middle of the second trimester most women say sayonara to puking in public.

WHAT IF MY WATER BREAKS IN PUBLIC?

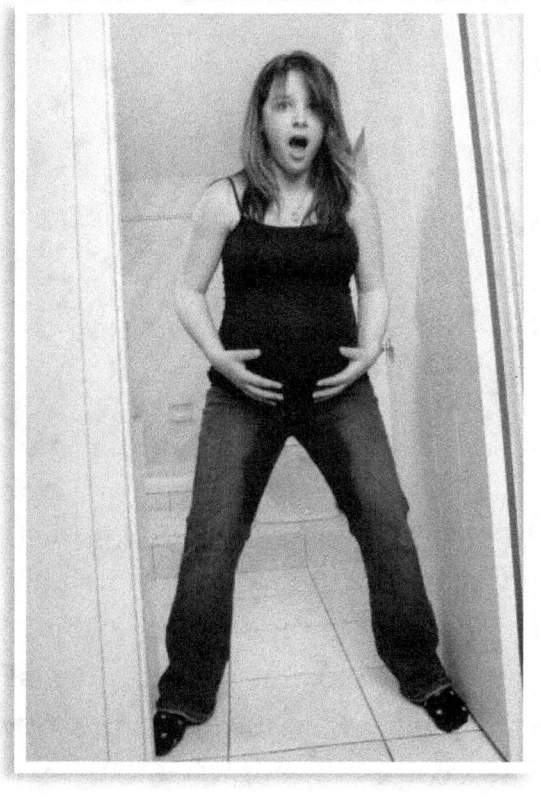

Another happy Hollywood scene is when the (impossibly svelte) pregnant heroine soaks the carpet with a whoosh of waters breaking. The truth is, this hardly ever happens. If your waters break in public, most women experience a slight trickle that is relatively easy to conceal in the rush to grab a ride to the hospital. Even if you do experience the gush, you've got bigger fish to fry than whatever the chap at the grocery counter thinks of you.

WHAT IS GOING ON WITH MY BELLY BUTTON?

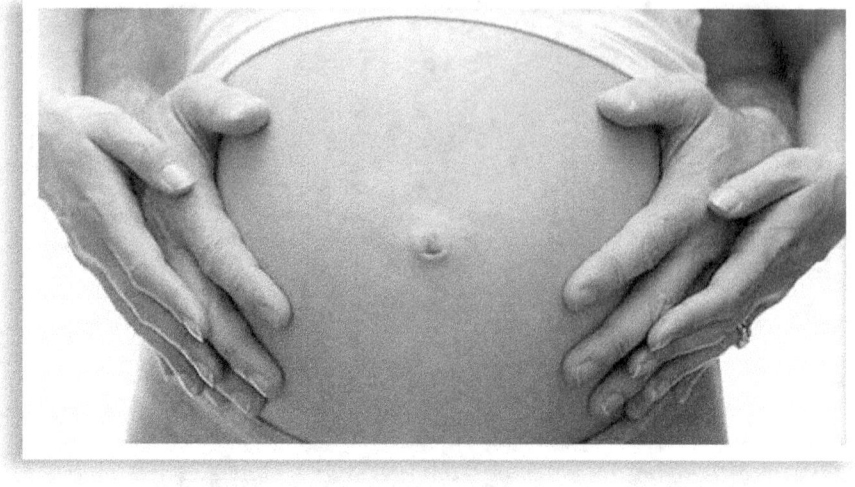

As your belly skin stretches, your navel is likely to go through many changes, up to and including becoming slightly distended beyond the stomach. This is completely normal, and will return to more or less normal when the baby's out and about. Make sure you moisturize plenty to help your skin recover in general.

WHAT ARE THESE RED MARKS SPREADING ACROSS MY BELLY?

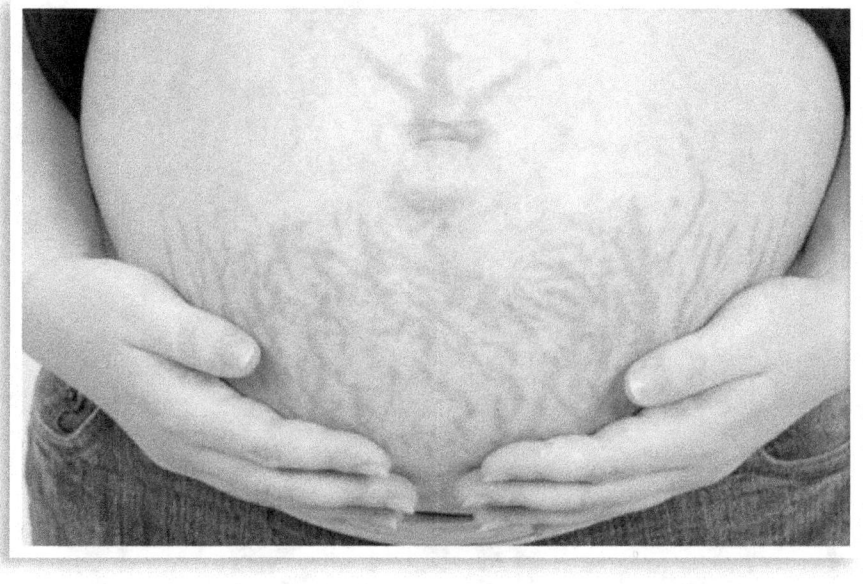

Stretch marks are a normal pregnancy side effect, but they can look particularly gruesome when the skin is still stretching. While you may not be able to fully disappear these insidious markings, you can buy a cream that's designed for reducing the appearance of stretch marks. Many women swear by good old-fashioned cocoa butter. This will also help with the itching. Even if the marks don't disappear, most of them will return to a color closely matching the skin around them once your skin has a chance to recover.

WHY DO I SMELL SO BAD?

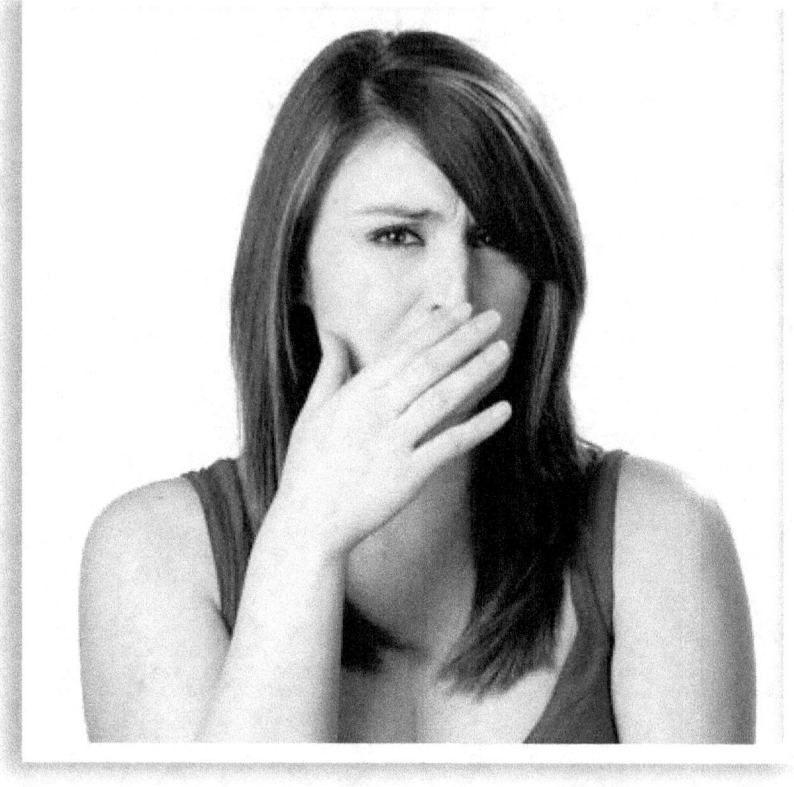

If you've noticed a distinct increase in your body odor, you can blame your hormones. In addition, you're probably sweating quite a bit, so up your shower frequency and stock up on your favorite deodorant.

I SWEAT ALL THE TIME, EVEN JUST SITTING AROUND. WHY?

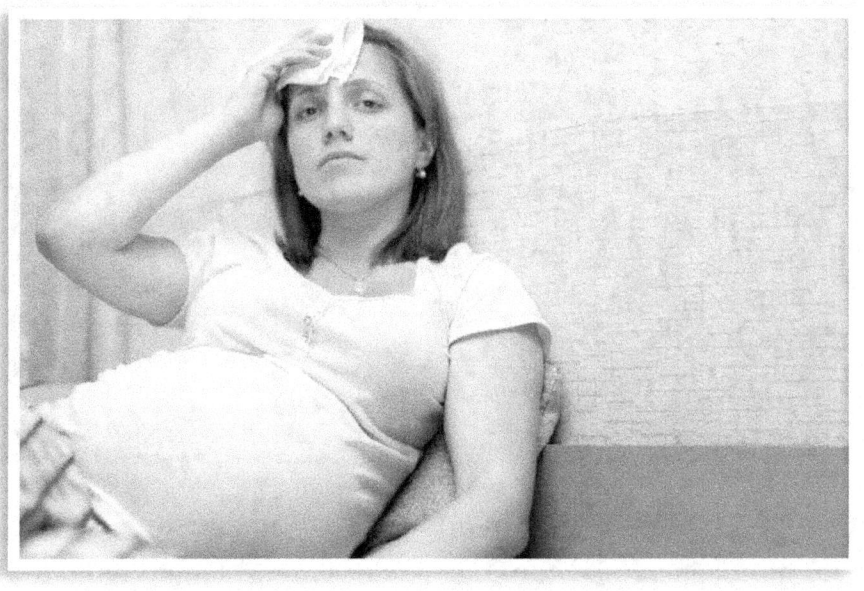

An increase in your blood flow as well as stress on your body can have you feeling the burn even when at rest. After all, your body is guiding the work of two humans now, so it's logical that you can run a bit hot. Make sure to drink plenty of water to replenish yourself, and maybe go swimming to cool down and get a great pregnancy approved workout.

WHY DOES EVERYTHING SMELL SO BAD?

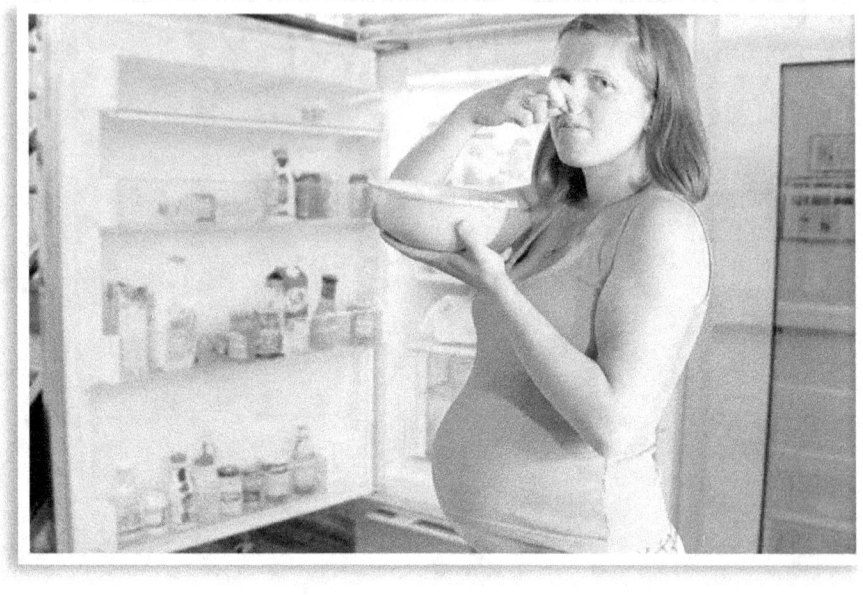

One of the most common and persistent signs of pregnancy is a heightened sense of smell. This means that especially during the first trimester you may be plugging your nose a lot. It can exacerbate nausea and other morning sickness symptoms, so be sure to keep mints or some other fresh scent handy. Feel free to request help from your spouse in the form of extra showers and not cooking pungent foods until you've got your gag reflex under control.

WHAT ON EARTH IS A MUCUS PLUG?

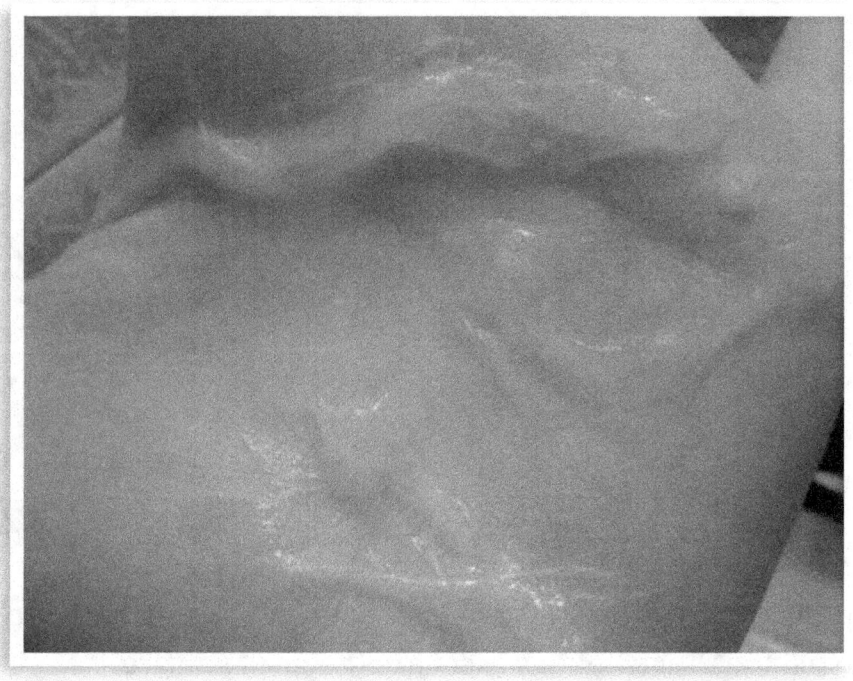

A mucus plug is just that: a protective plug of mucus that gathers on the cervix to protect the fetus inside from any nastiness. Yes, it is gross, and yes, it will probably make its exit in the latter weeks of pregnancy as baby prepares for the final descent. When it does, just flush it down the loo and keep on rolling. You can google what it will look like, but maybe in this case it's better to be surprised.

WHAT IF I POOP DURING DELIVERY?

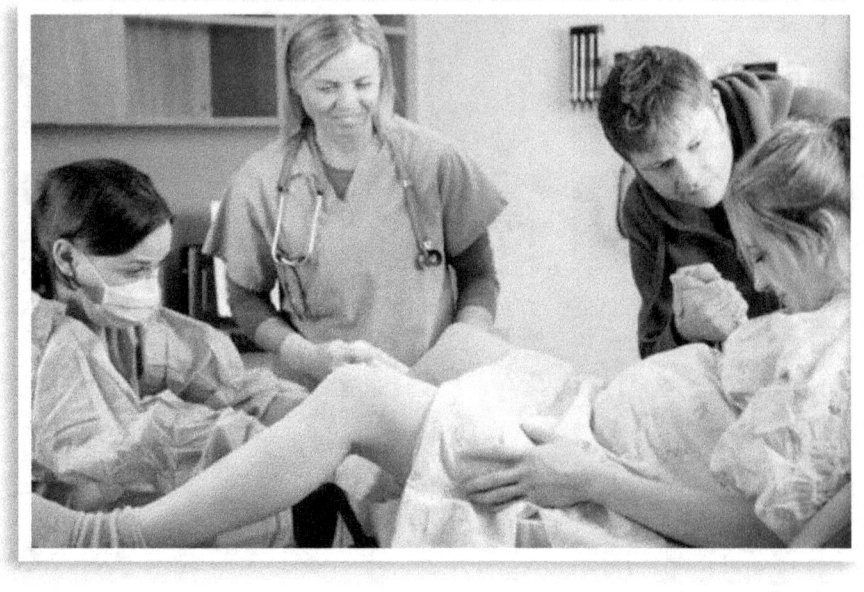

Many women do, as many of the same muscles you use to expel that huge holiday meal are the ones you are engaging to bring your little love into this world. The good news? Doctors see this all the time, and most of them won't even tell you that it happened. Nurses are trained to whisk it away without comment to minimize germs. Chalk it up to one of those things you didn't want to know anyway.

I'M SCARED ABOUT GIVING BIRTH!

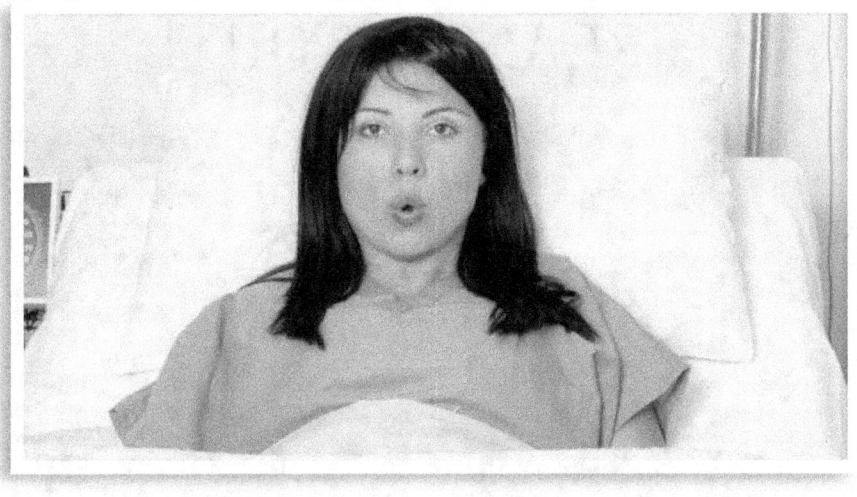

Of course you are! Everyone is to differing degrees. The best thing to do is avoid going in blind, so make a list of questions for your practitioner and pick up a few books to read. You can even put together a birth plan for what you would like to happen that day, and share it with your doctor and hospital staff. Things like this rarely go exactly as planned, but it will be good for you to go in knowing what may happen next.

I'VE GOT TO HAVE A CESAREAN SECTION, AND IT FREAKS ME OUT!

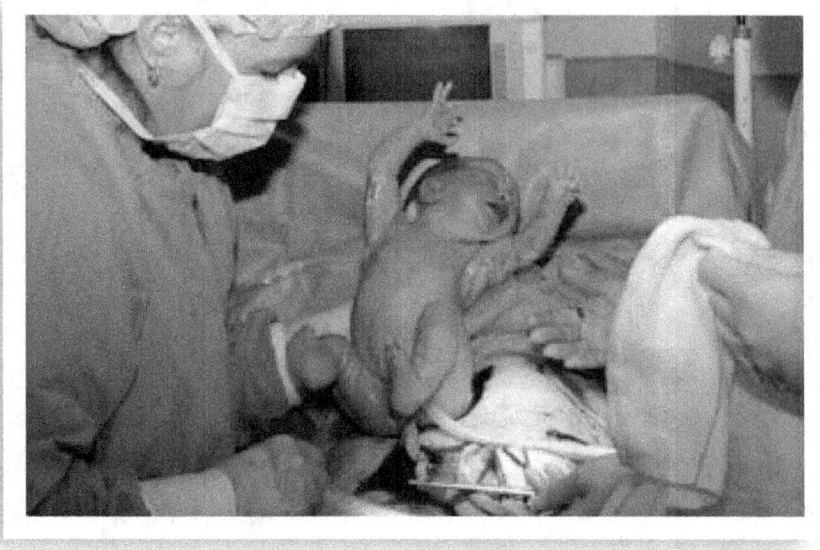

The c-section procedure is a common procedure that many doctors, including yours, have down to a science. Still, any time you will be having surgery, you should know exactly what's involved. In all but the most extreme cases, you will still be conscious for your child's birth. Also request a family-friendly procedure, where you get to hold the baby and stay with them through your recovery. Many hospitals are gravitating toward this type of procedure to the delight of c-section mothers everywhere.

IF I HAVE A C-SECTION, HOW BIG IS THE SCAR?

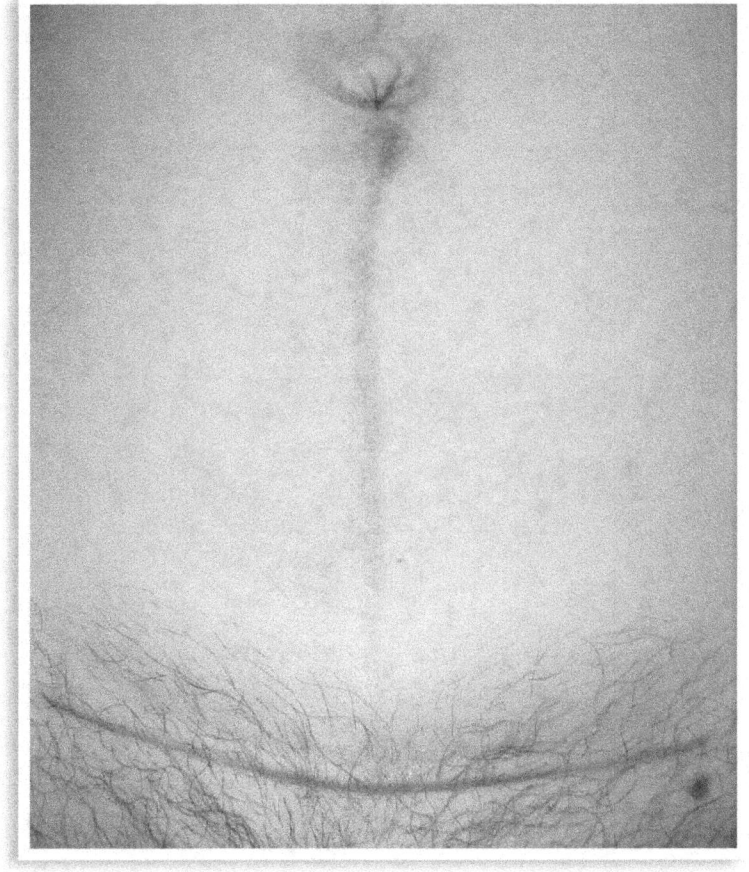

The scar you will have after a c-section depends on a number of factors, like your skin's capacity to regenerate, how big the incision needs to be, and how well you care for your sutures. There are also mitigating procedures like injections that your doctor can give you after you are sufficiently healed, which may minimize the appearance of your scar. The good news is that the scar will be so low that only your husband will ever have occasion to see it, and he has little right to complain.

CAN MY DOCTOR OR MIDWIFE TELL IF I'VE HAD SEX BEFORE LABOR?

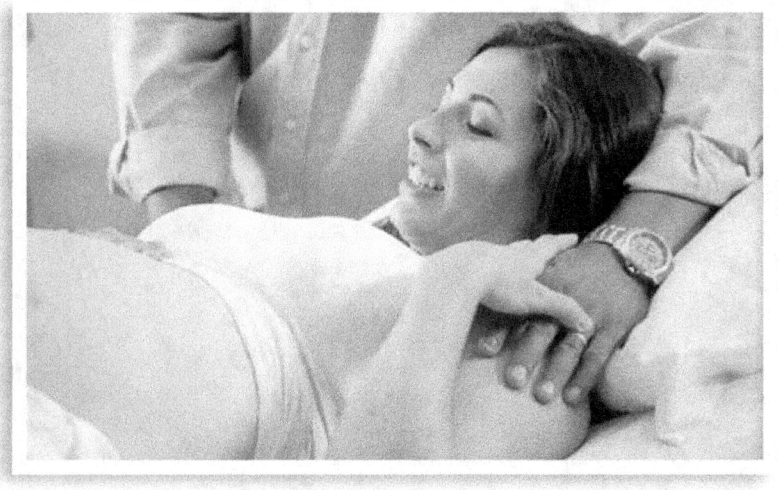

Since many women opt to try bringing on labor through sex, and this is actually quite effective at moving things along, you might think that the doctor will know they're sinking their fingers into a little love mixture. The truth is, between the waters and your normal vaginal discharge from pregnancy, there's very little chance that anyone will know the difference. Take a shower if you have the time or strength, and if not a little wipe can go a long way.

HOW MUCH BLOOD WILL COME OUT WITH BIRTH?

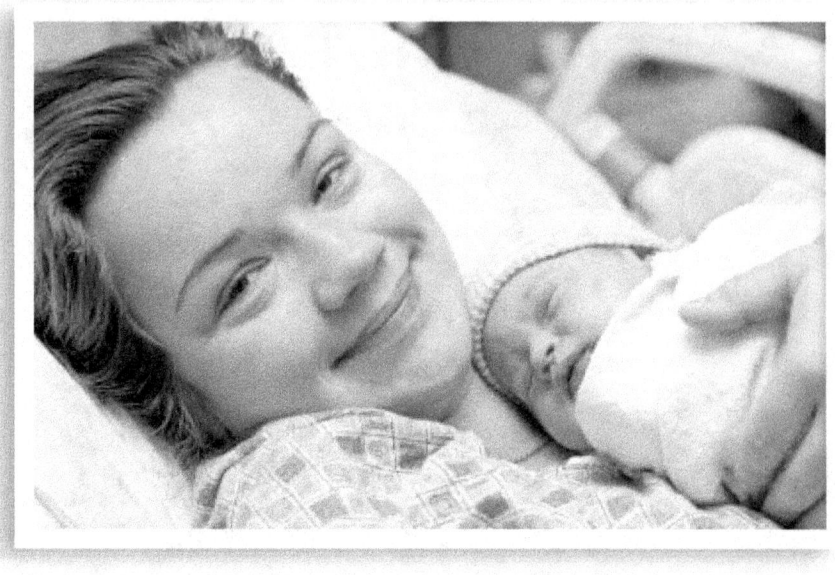

You might think that there's going to be a tsunami of blood and waters during birth, but in reality there is only a small amount of blood discharged. After you deliver your baby and the placenta, you can expect symptoms similar to a heavy period, which may last a few weeks. Make sure that you stock up on pads and comfortable panties for this time, as you'll need to stay away from tampons while you are healing.

WILL I BE ABLE TO USE THE LOO IN LABOR?

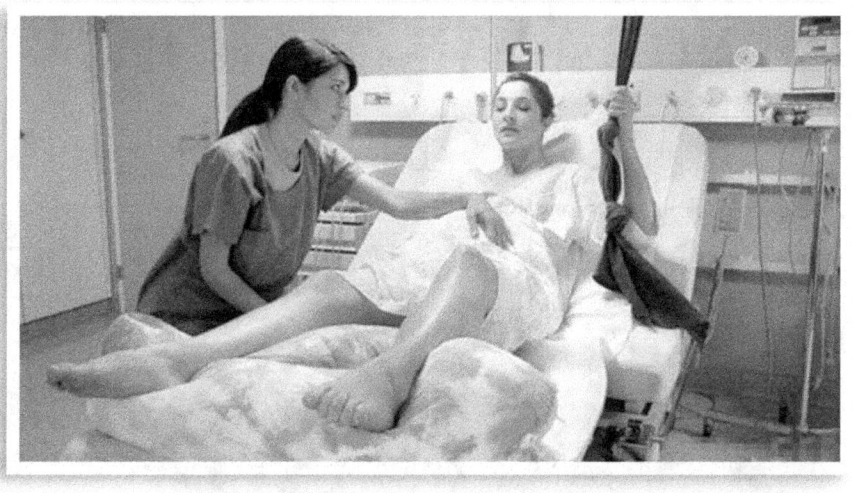

While it may seem that labor would block anything else from happening down there, it can actually be a rather long process during which you may have to answer the call of nature a few times. Until your contractions are coming hard and fast with no break, or they administer an epidural, you'll be able to take all the restroom breaks you need.

WHO IS GOING TO SEE MY PRIVATES DURING LABOR? I'M NOT A FAN OF SHOWING OFF.

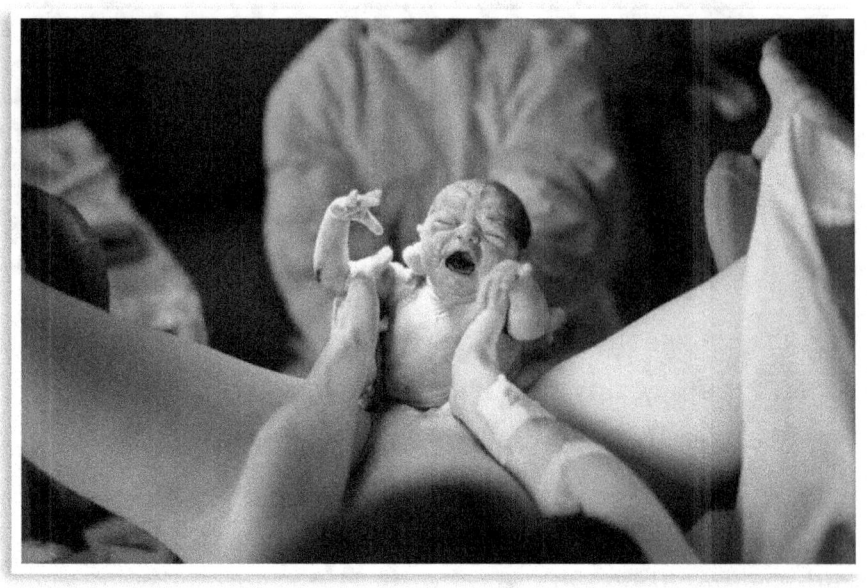

Talk to your doctor or midwife, but you usually have complete control over who's staring at your parts during the actual time. Only necessary medical staff need get up close and personal, and perhaps your partner. Everyone else is subject to your approval, so make it clear that the in-laws and your parents can wait until you're ready for visitors.

THERE'S A COATING ON MY BABY'S SKIN WHEN HE'S BORN?! GROSS!

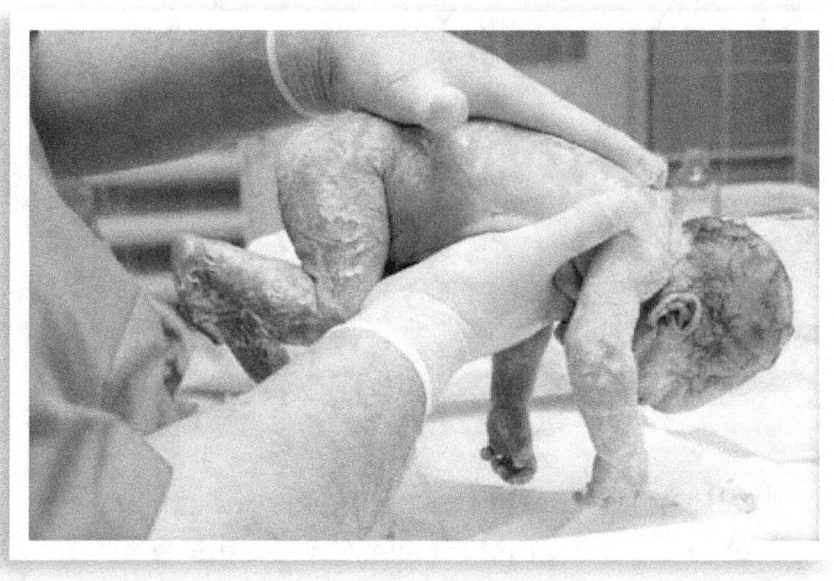

Vernix, a natural protective moisturizer that develops in utero to protect baby's skin, may still be present after birth. There's no rule about when to clean it off, but many women choose to let it absorb naturally into baby's skin.

HOW LONG UNTIL I CAN HAVE SEX AGAIN?

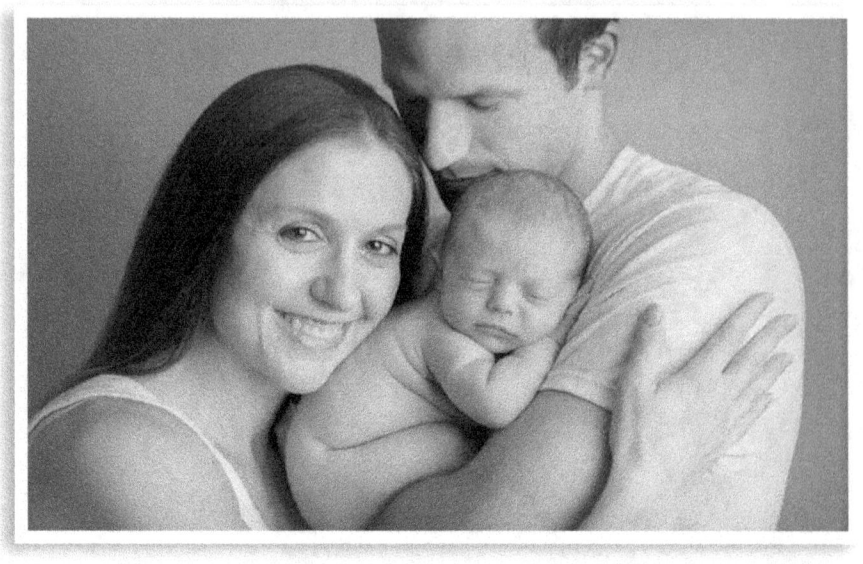

You should definitely find out from your doctor the minimum recommended recovery time after your particular birth. If there has been significant trauma to your lady bits, you may be required to wait as long as six weeks to hit it hard. However, you can always start slow with oral sex or mutual masturbation to gauge the field.

Thank You!

We hope you enjoyed the book! All pictures and words were lovingly put together by experts who really love what they do! We really hope you learned something new today!

We would really appreciate it, if you could PLEASE take the time to let us know how we're doing by leaving a review on the Amazon website. We appreciate any comments you may have – what you enjoyed about the book, what additions you would have liked to have seen and what you would like to see in future publications.

Any comments will help understand better what you and your kids most enjoy and allows us to better provide exactly what you want!

Thought Junction Publishing

A NOTE FROM THE WRITER

Sam's life revolves around her family, devoted mother of 3 - Noah (6), Oscar (3) and Poppy (11months) - she writes in a real way, aiming to answer the questions that other books don't cover, to fill in the blanks and inform parents and parents-to-be of the truth about raising children in the modern world.

Sam's writings emphasize that the readers are not alone - that there is a community of support available, and other people to talk to who can help, support and assist.

When she's not writing books, Sam is an advisor and avid blogger for Ideal Parent - http://ideal-parent.com - spreading support, care and advice across the web!

Join Sam on Ideal Parent and keep an eye out for her books - she's on a mission to help parents worldwide - join her and spread the word!

www.ingramcontent.com/pod-product-compliance
Lightning Source LLC
Chambersburg PA
CBHW071116280526
45787CB00003B/1064